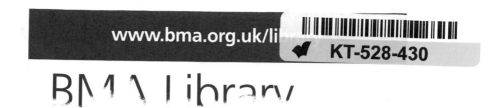
Get Through

MRCOG Part 2:
Short Answer Questions

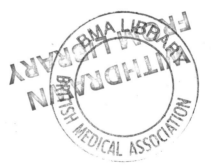

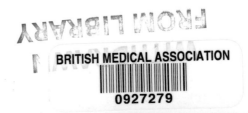

Get Through
MRCOG Part 2:
Short Answer Questions

Euan Kevelighan MB ChB FRCOG Dip Med Ed
Consultant Obstetrician and Gynaecologist, Singleton Hospital, Swansea;
All Wales Training Programme Director

Jeremy Gasson MB ChB FRCOG
Consultant Obstetrician and Gynaecologist, Singleton Hospital, Swansea;
Clinical Director, Women and Children's Services, ABM University NHS Trust

Makiya Ashraf MB BS MRCOG
Consultant Obstetrician and Gynaecologist, Royal Gwent Hospital, Gwent Healthcare
NHS Trust, Newport

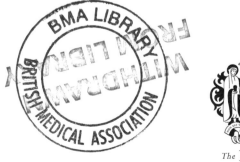

The ROYAL
SOCIETY *of*
MEDICINE
PRESS *Limited*

© 2009 Royal Society of Medicine Press Ltd

Published by the Royal Society of Medicine Press Ltd
1 Wimpole Street, London W1G 0AE, UK
Tel: +44 (0)20 7290 2921
Fax: +44 (0)20 7290 2929
E-mail: publishing@rsm.co.uk
Website: www.rsmpress.c.uk

British Library Cataloguing in Publication Data
A catalogue record for this book is available from the British Library

ISBN: 978-1-85315-856-8

Distribution in Europe and Rest of the World:
Marston Book Services Ltd
PO Box 269
Abingdon
Oxon OX14 4YN, UK
Tel: +44 (0)1235 465500
Fax: +44 (0)1235 465555
Email: direct.order@marston.co.uk

Distribution in the USA and Canada:
Royal Society of Medicine Press Ltd
c/o BookMasters Inc
30 Amberwood Parkway
Ashland, OH 44805, USA
Tel: +1 800 247 6553/+1 800 266 5564
Fax: +1 419 281 6883
Email: order@bookmasters.com

Distribution in Australia and New Zealand:
Elsevier Australia
30-52 Smidmore Street
Marrickville NSW 2204, Australia
Tel: +61 2 9517 8999
Fax: +61 2 9517 2249
Email: service@elsevier.com.au

Typeset by Techset Composition Limited, Salisbury, UK
Printed and bound in Great Britain by Bell & Bain, Glasgow

Contents

Dedication

To my wife for all her support and encouragement while writing this book. EHK
To my wife Helen and children, Katharine and David, for all their support. JG
To my family for their support. MA

Foreword

In 1996, there was a radical change in the MRCOG Part 2 examination. The old style of two obstetric and two gynaecology essays was replaced by the ten short answer questions. These have been shown to be much fairer and discriminate better between the good and the poor candidate. Over the succeeding years this new format has slowly developed to its present style, which continues to be an excellent test of understanding and thinking skills, of demonstrating an ability to select and organize ideas, and to test logical thinking.

This new book deserves to be popular. Its style is concise and easy to read, and it gives valuable assistance to those who find this element of the examination taxing.

Peter Bowen-Simpkins MA FRCOG FFFP
Immediate Past Honorary Treasurer, RCOG
Past Chairman, Short Answer Questions Subcommittee

Introduction

The MRCOG Part 2 examination has both a written and an oral component. It is designed to test the knowledge, understanding and skills of a candidate at the end of three years of registrar experience in UK practice (SpR year 3 or specialty registrar year 5).

The written component comprises:

- Two short answer question (SAQ) papers (formerly known as short essay questions).
- A multiple choice question (MCQ) paper of 225 questions.
- An extended matching question (EMQ) paper of 40 questions.

The candidate must pass the written examination in order to proceed to the oral examination. The written examination is marked out of 425 and the oral examination carries 200 marks. The mark from the written examination does *not* contribute to the score on the oral examination.

The marks for the written examination are made up as follows:

- MCQ paper – 225 questions worth 1 mark each = 225 marks (marked by computer).
- EMQ paper – 40 questions worth 1 mark each = 40 marks (marked by computer).
- SAQ paper – 8 questions, each marked out of 20 = 160 marks (marked by hand).

The EMQs test more complex understanding than the MCQs and are more valid and reliable. They assess the application of medical knowledge rather than simple factual recall. They were introduced into the Part 2 examination in September 2006. It is very likely the proportion of EMQs will increase and the numbers of MCQs decrease in future exams. Check the RCOG website (www.rcog.org.uk) for up-to-date information.

Blueprinting

All MRCOG examinations are subject to blueprinting. This ensures that no examination tests too much of one area and insufficient of another. The committee chairs (of MCQ, EMQ, SAQ and oral assessment) meet and confirm appropriate coverage of the syllabus by the forthcoming exam. An even spread of the curriculum is therefore tested.

Standard setting

All parts of the written and oral examination are subject to standard setting. The principle of standard setting is to set an objective pass mark for each exam. Standard setting ensures that the exam is fair and consistent and that the same standard is applied each time the Part 2 examination is held. Some exams will be easier than others and standard setting compensates for this by referencing the pass mark against a defined standard – 'criterion referencing'. Therefore the more difficult the exam, the lower the overall pass mark will be. Standard setting establishes the pass mark by determining the minimum amount of knowledge or skill required. It does not relate to the 'pass rate'. Standard setting is required to maintain the validity of the exam, to reassure the public and to counter legal challenges.

For SAQs limen (Latin for threshold) referencing is used. This technique relies on the difference between a clear pass and a clear fail answer. A group of examiners read a single SAQ and are asked to classify which answers are clear passes and which are clear fails. The answers where the examiners cannot decide if they are a clear pass or a clear fail (the borderline group) are disregarded for standard setting. Standard setting is completely separate from and completed prior to the marking of the papers.

The pass mark for each SAQ varies to reflect its difficulty. Typically a pass mark ranges between 10 and 13 (out of 20) and is determined by standard setting. (Occasionally a pass mark may be below 10 or above 13.) Approximately 25% of candidates pass the written examination and over 75% of those who attend for the oral examination will pass.

Short answer questions (SAQs)

There are two papers, each with four questions. Both papers last 1 hour and 45 minutes (105 minutes); therefore you will have approximately 26 minutes for each question. Paper 1 has four SAQs primarily relating to obstetrics, including labour ward practice and prenatal diagnosis. Paper 2 has four gynaecological SAQs and may include areas such as screening and disease prevention.

Each question is marked out of 20. No half marks are permitted. Up to four marks can be deducted for dangerous clinical practice and a further two marks for persistent factual errors.

Recently, SAQs have been modified. Most questions have three or four parts. One sheet of A4 is provided by the RCOG for each question. Each question (or part of a question) is followed by a finite space in which the candidate inserts an answer. Both sides of the one sheet of A4 may be used. No extra paper is provided or permitted for answers. Answers must be placed in the correct space for each sub-division of a question. The candidate must not write outside the designated areas, and any information written there will be ignored and attract no marks.

Some coloured paper is provided on which to make notes. We strongly suggest you use this for your essay plan.

The SAQs assess your critical understanding of the practice of obstetrics and gynaecology in the UK – typically to the level of a third-year registrar (SpR3/ST5). They typically ask you to 'describe', 'define', 'explain', 'identify', 'justify', 'compare and contrast', give 'pros and cons', or 'critically evaluate'; most relate to patient management.

It is vitally important you write concisely and legibly, in the space provided.

Preparation for the SAQ examination

There are many resources available. We strongly suggest you focus on the journals and resources which are most likely to give you the highest yield of potential exam questions. After each answer we include reference(s) that we used to construct the sample answers and which can be used to obtain further information. You do not need to quote references in the actual examination.

We believe the following texts are essential reading.

1. *The Obstetrician and Gynaecologist (TOG)*. Published four times a year by the RCOG, *TOG* is the RCOG's journal of continuing professional development. It contains up-to-date, peer-reviewed articles. Frequently, such articles are the basis of SAQs. *TOG* is available online at www.rcog.org.uk/togonline.
2. 'Green-Top Guidelines'. Published by the RCOG, these documents provide practice recommendations for many areas of clinical practice. They are reviewed and updated usually every three years. The guidelines are concise and very useful for answering SAQs, as well as helpful for objective structured clinical examinations (OSCEs), EMQs and MCQs. See www.rcog.org.uk/index.asp?PageID=1042.
3. *Obstetrics, Gynaecology and Reproductive Medicine* (formerly called *Current Obstetrics and Gynaecology*). Published monthly by Elsevier, this British journal covers the Part 2 MRCOG syllabus every three years. Each issue contains review articles. Each month a section is devoted to self-assessment, which includes MCQs, EMQs and frequently a worked example of the newer-type SAQs, with a suggested marking system. Practise these questions and see your confidence grow. See www.sciencedirect.com/science/journal/17517214.
4. *BJOG: An International Journal of Obstetrics and Gynaecology*. Owned by the RCOG, this journal is published monthly by Blackwell Publishing. Commentaries, review articles, short communications and correspondence (the letter section) often contain nuggets of information useful for answering SAQs. See www.blackwellpublishing.com/bjog.
5. The 'MRCOG and Beyond' series. Published by RCOG Press, this series is well written, concise, up-to-date and useful for answering SAQs. For all the current titles see www.rcog.org.uk/index.asp.

We would suggest you review:

- All the Green-Top Guidelines (there are now more than 50).
- The most recent three years of *Obstetrics, Gynaecology and Reproductive Medicine* (i.e. one full cycle of the MRCOG Part 2 syllabus).
- The last two years of *TOG* and *BJOG*.

You will notice we have used many Green-Top Guidelines, *TOG* and *Obstetrics, Gynaecology and Reproductive Medicine* articles as sources for the 100 questions in this book. We believe they provide an excellent resource of likely topics for SAQs, MCQs, EMQs and OSCEs.

When the examiners are setting the questions, they look for ideas in the current literature. They tend to set the questions about 12 months prior to the exam. Frequently, the topics are new to the examination, although old important questions (e.g. on pre-eclampsia or antepartum haemorrhage) will be refined and reused.

How to write excellent answers to SAQs

It is essential to practise SAQs so that you learn to:

- Write concisely and legibly.
- Answer the questions/sub-division of the questions actually asked.
- Keep to time (26 minutes per question).

You must write in sentences. Lists, short notes, bullet points and abbreviations will result in you being marked down. The English needs to be understandable to the examiner. Marks are not lost for spelling mistakes or use of the wrong tense, for example. However, practising SAQs and having them corrected by a colleague who writes correct English will help to eliminate these errors.

You may find it helpful to underline the main point in each paragraph. Use a ruler for this.

Use a biro or ink pen to write your answers to the SAQs. Bring your own.

Do not write an introduction to the SAQ unless it actually answers part of the question.

Be selective in what you write. Most marks are gained in the first few sentences of your answer and writing information irrelevant to the question will gain no marks and use up valuable space. In the event of mistakes, you will not be given any replacement paper so think very carefully before writing.

Read the question very carefully *twice*. Identify the key words (you can underline them in the question) and write a short essay plan (take 2–5 minutes for this) on the rough coloured paper provided. Prioritize your points. If you do not write an essay plan you will likely forget something important or remember it later and have no space left in which to write it down.

When you read a question, look at the number of marks allocated to each of its parts. This informs you how much time you should give this sub-division of the answer. Most questions have three or four parts. Some parts are worth 7 to 10 marks, while others may only attract 1 or 2 marks. The total number of marks per question will always add up to 20.

Stick rigidly to your time of 26 minutes per question. Do not be tempted to spend more time on questions that you know you can answer better.

Attempt all questions (four on each paper). Any question unanswered is scored 0 out of 20. It is very unlikely you will pass the written examination if you receive no marks on one of the eight SAQs.

Answer the questions based on good evidence where possible. Your answers will depend on your clinical experience and your ability to justify or explain the patient management you propose. Most marks are given for critical evaluation; for example, why you request a particular test or investigation for a specific patient.

Most candidates who fail the SAQs do so because:

- They lack the clinical experience required to answer the questions, or
- They do not answer the question asked.

Most candidates tend to answer the SAQs in the third person (e.g. 'the patient should be reassured', 'this investigation should be performed'). Since many questions ask 'What would you do?', it is often more appropriate to answer using the first person, i.e. 'I would . . .'. Also it is often helpful in answering SAQs to imagine the patient with the problem sitting in front of you in the clinic – what would you say and do?

Remember, practice makes perfect. Good luck.

Summary

1. Read the question twice.
2. Make an essay plan on the coloured paper provided (2–5 minutes).
3. Answer the question asked (not the question you might like to answer).
4. Be concise.
5. Write legibly.
6. Move on to the next question after 26 minutes.

Do not

1. Use a pencil.
2. Write using lists, bullet points and abbreviations.

Getting the most out of this book

This book is divided into two sections. The first gives 27 SAQs and suggested answers on obstetrics and 25 SAQs and suggested answers on gynaecology. The second section presents further SAQs but set out in the format of the MRCOG Part 2 exam. There are six such practice exams. These comprise two papers, covering obstetrics and gynaecology respectively, of four questions each. There are, thus, 100 questions in total in the book, which will give a sound foundation for the exam itself.

Many suggested answers have extra information included which is not directly relevant to answer the question or sub-division of the question. Such additional information is enclosed in square brackets, '[...]', and is provided to enhance your understanding; it may also be useful if a similar question appears as an SAQ.

We hope you enjoy and benefit from this book. We suggest you read the question and then, before reading the answer, close the book. Write an essay plan (2–5 minutes) and then write your short answer. Stop after 26 minutes (including the essay preparation time). Mark your question against our suggested marking scheme. It is not possible to say exactly what mark is a pass (due to standard setting, as explained above), although it tends to be approximately 10–13 out of 20.

Finally, remember that practice makes perfect.

We would like to hear from users. Please send any feedback, suggestions or comments to publishing@rsm.ac.uk.

Further reading

1. Examination section of the RCOG website, www.rcog.org.uk/index.asp?PageID=36.
2. Fogarty P. Mock MRCOG Part II short answer question. *Obstetrics, Gynaecology and Reproductive Medicine* 2008; **18**: 80–1.
3. Ledger W, Murphy M, Hodges P. Format and structure of the Part 2 MRCOG examination. *Obstetrics, Gynaecology and Reproductive Medicine* 2007; **17**: 62–4.
4. Ledger WL, Murphy M, eds. *The MRCOG: A Guide to the Examination* (3rd edition). London: RCOG Press, 2008.

SECTION I
PRACTICE QUESTIONS

1.1.1 Shoulder dystocia

A What is the incidence of shoulder dystocia (SD) and what factors are associated with it? (5 marks)

B Discuss how you would manage a case of shoulder dystocia. (10 marks)

C What are the maternal and neonatal complications of this obstetric emergency? (5 marks)

1.1.2 Group B streptococcal (GBS) disease

A woman attending the booking clinic is very anxious, as she lost her last baby at one week of age from early-onset Group B streptococcal (GBS) disease.

A What are the risk factors for GBS disease? (5 marks)

B How should this woman's pregnancy and delivery be managed? (8 marks)

C What are the arguments against universal screening and treatment in the UK? (7 marks)

1.1.3 Uterine inversion

You are called to attend a collapsed patient on the labour ward.

A What is the estimated incidence of uterine inversion and what findings are associated with this condition? (4 marks)

B What are the symptoms and signs of uterine inversion? (5 marks)

C You diagnose uterine inversion in this case. What is your initial management? (6 marks)

D What are your options for replacement of the uterus? (5 marks)

1.1.4 Cord prolapse

A Define cord prolapse and outline the difference between it and cord presentation. (2 marks)

B What is the incidence of cord prolapse and discuss the antenatal (non-procedural) risk factors associated with it? (8 marks)

C What procedures are associated with an increased risk of cord prolapse? (5 marks)

D What would you advise a paramedic in the community to do when faced with a cord prolapse prior to transfer to hospital? (5 marks)

1.1.5   Twin–twin transfusion

A 35-year-old woman attends the booking clinic at 12 weeks' gestation and ultrasound scan reveals a twin pregnancy.

A   What are the important features of this pregnancy on ultrasound scan and why? (6 marks)

B   How should her antenatal care be planned? (7 marks)

C   What is twin-to-twin transfusion syndrome (TTTS) and how is it managed? (7 marks)

1.1.6   Gestational diabetes

A primigravid woman at 28 weeks' gestation is referred from midwifery-led care with an ultrasound diagnosis of a macrosomic fetus but with no other abnormalities.

A   What are the risk factors for gestational diabetes mellitus (GDM) and how is it diagnosed? (7 marks)

B   If GDM is confirmed, how will her delivery be planned? (7 marks)

C   What postnatal care and advice should she be given? (6 marks)

1.1.7   Non-immune hydrops

A 24-year-old woman who is 25 weeks' pregnant contacts her community midwife as her daughter has just been diagnosed with 'slapped cheek' syndrome. She is concerned about the potential effects of her daughter's illness on her pregnancy. The midwife contacts the hospital for advice.

A   What advice should the patient receive at this stage? (6 marks)

B   Two weeks later this woman's fetus develops non-immune hydrops (NIH). How should this be investigated? (9 marks)

C   Assuming the NIH is due to infection following her daughter's 'slapped cheek' syndrome, how should this be managed antenatally? (5 marks)

1.1.8   Thyroid disease

A woman attends the antenatal clinic at 20 weeks' gestation. Investigations show she has thyrotoxicosis due to Graves' disease.

A   Identify three of the more discriminatory features of hyperthyroidism in pregnancy. (3 marks)

B   How is thyrotoxicosis caused by Graves' disease diagnosed and what are the risks to this pregnancy? (8 marks)

C   Outline your management of this woman's thyrotoxicosis. (7 marks)

D   What are the indications for thyroidectomy in pregnancy? (2 marks)

3   **1.1.9   Obesity in pregnancy**

A chronically morbidly obese patient undergoes emergency caesarean section (CS) at full cervical dilatation.

A   What difficulties might the obstetrician encounter during CS? (5 marks)

B   Describe possible postoperative complications and how you might reduce them. (11 marks)

C   What pre-existing diseases might a patient who is chronically morbidly obese have at booking for antenatal care? (4 marks)

3   **1.1.10   Cardiopulmonary arrest**

You are the registrar on call for the labour ward and you are called to attend a collapsed patient in triage who was admitted at 34 weeks' gestation with a swollen left leg.

A   What is your initial management of this situation? (3 marks)

B   How would you diagnose a cardiopulmonary arrest? (4 marks)

C   Assuming that this patient has had a cardiopulmonary arrest, describe how you would perform basic life support. (6 marks)

D   How would you use an automated external defibrillator (AED) and what are the two shockable rhythms? (6 marks)

E   What is the likely diagnosis? (1 mark)

2   **1.1.11   Vaginal birth after caesarean section (VBAC)**

A 32-year-old woman in her second pregnancy attends the antenatal clinic at 24 weeks' gestation to discuss the method of delivery for her current pregnancy. She had an emergency caesarean section for fetal distress at 6 cm last time.

A   What are the contraindications to vaginal birth after caesarean section (VBAC) in general? (5 marks)

B   Outline the risks and benefits of VBAC. (11 marks)

C   What intrapartum support would you plan for this labour? (4 marks)

2   **1.1.12   Ovarian cysts in pregnancy**

A 34-year-old woman is seen in the antenatal clinic with an asymptomatic adnexal mass identified on ultrasound scan (USS) at 11 weeks' gestation.

A   Give four causes of an adnexal mass in pregnancy. (Assume the pregnancy is intrauterine.) (4 marks)

B   In what percentage of pregnancies are adnexal masses reported on USS? (1 mark)

C   Discuss the management of this case, assuming the adnexal mass was ovarian. (13 marks)

D   Is there a role for assessment of tumour markers in ovarian cysts in pregnancy? (2 marks)

1.1.13 Alcohol in pregnancy

A 36-year-old attending the antenatal booking clinic smells of alcohol. On questioning she admits to regular binge drinking (>5 drinks at one session) and a heavy alcohol intake for the past two years.

A What advice would you give this woman? (7 marks)

B Outline the potential risks to this pregnancy related to her alcohol intake. (9 marks)

C What are the diagnostic criteria for fetal alcohol syndrome (FAS)? (4 marks)

1.1.14 Preterm premature rupture of membranes

A 37-year-old primigravida with a pregnancy from in vitro fertilization and normal antenatal progress presents to the antenatal day unit (ANDU) at 26 weeks' gestation with a history suggestive of ruptured membranes.

A Outline your immediate management. (10 marks)

B Assuming rupture of membranes is confirmed, describe your subsequent management. (10 marks)

1.1.15 Consent to caesarean section

You are the registrar on the labour ward. You are asked to obtain Mrs Smith's consent for her elective caesarean section for breech presentation.

A Describe to Mrs Smith (in non-medical language) what the procedure involves. (7 marks)

B What are the alternatives to delivery by caesarean section for Mrs Smith and what are the risks? (8 marks)

C What are the serious risks of caesarean section you would discuss with Mrs Smith? (5 marks)

1.1.16 Renal disease in pregnancy

A primigravida attends booking clinic at eight weeks' gestation and gives a history of polycystic kidney disease.

A Outline the relevant management at this booking visit? (5 marks)

B She is diagnosed as having moderate renal impairment. What specific risks does she have during this pregnancy? (4 marks)

C How will you plan the management of her pregnancy? (5 marks)

D At 28 weeks' gestation she presents with fever, loin pain and rigors. A provisional diagnosis of acute pyelonephritis is made. How should this be managed? (6 marks)

1.1.17 Cardiac disease in pregnancy

A 22-year-old primigravida attends the booking clinic at 14 weeks' gestation. She has recently arrived in the UK from Pakistan and gives a history of rheumatic fever in childhood. On examination she is found to be mildly dyspnoeic.

A What is the most likely diagnosis? (1 mark)

B Outline appropriate antenatal management. (7 marks)

C How should her delivery be managed? (9 marks)

D How should she be managed in the puerperium? (3 marks)

1.1.18 Screening

A What are the principles of screening? (10 marks)

B What serum screening tests are available for Down syndrome? What are the detection rates, assuming a 5% false positive rate? (6 marks)

C Discuss the combined test for Down syndrome. (4 marks)

1.1.19 Blood transfusion in obstetrics

A How may the risk of blood transfusion be reduced in the obstetric population? (8 marks)

B Outline four risks of blood transfusion. (4 marks)

C Discuss four blood components that may be required in the treatment of massive obstetric haemorrhage and describe in what clinical situation they may be used. (8 marks)

1.1.20 Fetus small for gestational age

A primigravid patient is referred by her midwife to the antenatal assessment unit at 32 weeks' gestation with reduced fetal movements and a symphyseal–fundal height of 26 cm. An ultrasound scan suggests a fetus small for gestational age (SGA).

A What are the causes of a fetus being small for gestational age (SGA)? (7 marks)

B Outline appropriate antenatal care for the rest of this pregnancy. (8 marks)

C Identify the potential short- and long-term sequelae of a SGA fetus. (5 marks)

1.1.21 Genital herpes

A primigravida presents to the antenatal clinic at 36 weeks' gestation with a primary episode of genital herpes (GH).

A Justify your management. (10 marks)

B Another patient attends your antenatal clinic later the same day at term with a recurrent episode of genital herpes. Outline appropriate management. (7 marks)

C How may genital herpes infection in pregnancy be reduced? (2 marks)

D How may postnatal transmission of the herpes simplex virus (HSV) to the neonate be prevented? (1 mark)

1.1.22 Massive obstetric haemorrhage

A Define massive obstetric haemorrhage and state what the difficulty is in clinical practice with this definition. (2 marks)

B Apart from uterine atony, give two other major causes of obstetric haemorrhage. (2 marks)

C How do you define shock and what are the maternal signs of it? (5 marks)

D How would you treat a woman having an atonic postpartum haemorrhage (PPH), following active management of the third stage? (11 marks)

1.1.23 Sickle cell disease in pregnancy

A 28-year-old woman with sickle cell disease attends your clinic, as she plans to start a family.

A What preconceptual evaluation is important? (5 marks)

B Outline the risks of sickle cell disease in pregnancy. (6 marks)

C How should her antenatal care be managed? (9 marks)

1.1.24 Thromboprophylaxis

A 27-year-old woman attends the antenatal booking clinic at 10 weeks' gestation. She gives a history of having had a deep vein thrombosis (DVT) when she returned from a holiday in Thailand.

A If she has no other risk factors, what counselling would you give her regarding thromboprophylaxis? (5 marks)

B Discuss pre-existing risk factors for venous thromboembolism in pregnancy. (8 marks)

C Under what other circumstances should antenatal thromboprophylaxis be considered? (7 marks)

1.1.25 Symphysis pubis diastasis

A patient at 34 weeks' gestation comes to see you in the antenatal clinic complaining of symptoms suggestive of symphysis pubis diastasis.

A What is the aetiology of this condition? (5 marks)

B What is the usual clinical presentation? (3 marks)

C What are the clinical signs and how is the diagnosis confirmed? (4 marks)

D What are the management options? (5 marks)

E How would you plan delivery of the baby? (3 marks)

1.1.26 Confidential enquiry into maternal and child health

The most recent report from the Confidential Enquiry into Maternal and Child Health (CEMACH), that for 2003–5, was published in December 2007.

A Outline three differences from previous reports. (3 marks)

B Discuss four objectives of the report. (4 marks)

C Define direct, indirect, coincidental and late deaths. Which type of death was the highest for this triennium? (5 marks)

D What were the commonest causes of direct and indirect death in this report? (2 marks)

E The maternal mortality rate has not declined since the mid-1980s. What factors have contributed to this lack of decline in deaths? (6 marks)

2 **1.1.27 Twin pregnancy**

The incidence of twin pregnancy has gradually increased over the last decade.

A What complications are associated with twin pregnancies? (10 marks)

B What are the difficulties with antenatal screening for trisomy 21 in twin pregnancies? (5 marks)

C What complications are associated with the intrauterine death of one twin? (5 marks)

Obstetrics: Answers

1.1.1 Shoulder dystocia

A What is the incidence of shoulder dystocia (SD) and what factors are associated with it? (5 marks)

B Discuss how you would manage a case of shoulder dystocia. (10 marks)

C What are the maternal and neonatal complications of this obstetric emergency? (5 marks)

Key words in the question

- Incidence, shoulder dystocia, factors.
- Management.
- Maternal, neonatal complications.

Essay plan

A

- State the incidence and discuss the aetiological factors of shoulder dystocia.

B

- Methodically outline the management of shoulder dystocia using the HELPERR mnemonic.

C

- Discuss the types of maternal and neonatal morbidity and their incidence.

Suggested answer

A

Shoulder dystocia occurs in approximately 6/1000 deliveries (1). Aetiological factors include those which exist pre-labour and those which occur or become apparent during labour. Pre-labour factors include previous shoulder dystocia, and recurrence rates are quoted as being between 1% and 16%. Fetal macrosomia is also associated, although it is not necessarily a good predictor, as half of the incidences of shoulder dystocia occur in babies with a birthweight less than 4 kg. Maternal body mass index (BMI) of greater than 30 kg/m² is also a risk factor. Diabetes mellitus and its association with both macrosomia and high maternal BMI is also a factor (2). Intrapartum factors include induction of labour and prolongation of both first and second stages. The use of oxytocin and a secondary arrest also make shoulder dystocia more likely. All these factors have a low positive predictive value, both singly and in combination, demonstrating that shoulder dystocia is an unpredictable and therefore unpreventable event (2).

B

Even though the factors above have a poor positive predictive value, experienced obstetricians should make themselves available on the labour ward when a shoulder dystocia may be anticipated (1).

Following diagnosis, the HELPERR mnemonic should be used. This stands for:

H – call for Help. All available staff should be called, including senior obstetrician, anaesthetist, midwife, theatre staff and porters (1).

E – the patient should be evaluated for an Episiotomy. This involves positioning of the woman in lithotomy to perform the episiotomy, thus allowing the accoucher access into the vagina for subsequent manoeuvres (1).

L – the woman's Legs should then be placed in McRoberts' position, which is flexion and abduction of the maternal hips, positioning the maternal thighs onto her abdomen. This increases the lumbosacral angle and is the single most effective manoeuvre, with delivery rates as high as 90% (1).

P – suprapubic Pressure, to the back of the fetal shoulder, is employed to cause reduction of the bisacromial diameter and to rotate the anterior shoulder to the oblique position, causing it to slip under the symphysis pubis and therefore facilitate delivery (1).

E – if this is unsuccessful, then the vagina is Entered to allow internal manipulations such as the Woods screw and reverse screw manoeuvres designed to rotate the anterior shoulder from under the symphysis pubis to allow delivery (1).

R – if the screw manoeuvres are unsuccessful, then the posterior arm may be Removed to allow delivery of the baby directly or via rotation of the fetal trunk using the arm (1).

R – Rolling of the woman onto all fours may at this stage cause displacement of the shoulder allowing delivery (1).

If the baby is still not delivered, then consideration should be given for symphysiotomy (division of the symphyseal ligament) with support of the maternal legs or Zavanelli's manoeuvre, which involves replacement of the fetal head into the vagina and delivery via caesarean section (2).

C

Maternal morbidities associated with shoulder dystocia are postpartum haemorrhage (11%) and fourth-degree tears (3.8%), and their incidence appears to be unchanged by the manoeuvres employed (2).

Symphysiotomy can cause trauma to the maternal urethra and bladder (1).

Brachial plexus injuries such as Erb's palsy occur in up to 16% of cases and can cause long-term problems in 10% of these babies (1).

If the baby remains undelivered for more than four minutes, brain damage or death may occur (1).

Further reading

Royal College of Obstetricians and Gynaecologists. *Shoulder Dystocia*. Green-Top Guideline No. 42. London: RCOG, December 2005.

1.1.2 Group B streptococcal (GBS) disease

A woman attending the booking clinic is very anxious, as she lost her last baby at one week of age from early-onset Group B streptococcal (GBS) disease.

A   What are the risk factors for GBS disease? (5 marks)

B   How should this woman's pregnancy and delivery be managed? (8 marks)

C   What are the arguments against universal screening and treatment in the UK? (7 marks)

Key words in the question

- Booking clinic, anxious, lost her last baby, GBS disease.
- Risk factors, GBS disease.
- How, pregnancy, delivery, managed.
- Arguments against universal screening.

Essay plan

A

- History previously affected baby, bacteriuria, preterm labour, prolonged ROM, pyrexia.

B

- No screening or antenatal treatment.
- Intrapartum antibiotic prophylaxis.
- Treat the neonate until blood culture results are available.
- Breast-feeding OK.

C

- No definite evidence of benefit from screening.
- Risks of widespread use of antibiotics and anaphylaxis.
- Financial implications on the service.

Suggested answer

A

The recognized risk factors for Group B streptococcal (GBS) disease are: a history of a previously affected baby (1); GBS bacteriuria detected in the current pregnancy or GBS colonization at term (1); preterm labour (1); prolonged rupture of membranes (1); and pyrexia during labour (1).

B

Routine screening is not recommended for antenatal GBS carriage (1). Even if this woman has GBS detected antenatally, treatment with antibiotics is not recommended, as it does not reduce the likelihood of GBS colonization at term (1). However, as this woman has a recognized risk factor for early-onset neonatal GBS disease (previous child dying of GBS infection), intrapartum prophylaxis against this condition should be offered and documented antenatally (1). Intrapartum antibiotic prophylaxis should be started as soon as labour is diagnosed (1). Intravenous penicillin at an initial dose of 3 g followed by 1.5 g every four hours until delivery is recommended (1). Clindamycin 900 mg intravenously every eight hours is given in patients allergic to penicillin (1). Since her previous child was affected by GBS, the newborn baby should either be closely observed for at least 12 hours or have blood cultures taken and be treated with antibiotics until the culture results are available (1).

As breast-feeding does not increase the risk of neonatal disease, the woman can be reassured regarding this method of feeding (1).

C

There is no strong evidence to suggest that screening for GBS has any impact on neonatal sepsis (1). Although intrapartum antibiotic prophylaxis has been shown to significantly reduce early-onset GBS disease, there can be risks associated with this (1). The risk of severe anaphylaxis from penicillin has been estimated at 1/10,000 and fatal anaphylaxis as 1/100,000 women treated (1). If a bacteriological screening programme were introduced in the UK, approximately 30% of the pregnant population would receive antibiotic prophylaxis and this might result in two deaths per year from anaphylaxis (1). The use of antibiotic prophylaxis may affect neonatal faecal flora, with a subsequent impact on immune development and later allergy (1). The widespread use of antibiotics contributes to the development of resistant organisms (1). This large cohort of pregnant women needing antibiotic prophylaxis during labour would also have an effect on the way our maternity services are currently delivered and would have financial implications (1).

Further reading

Royal College of Obstetricians and Gynaecologists. *Prevention of Early Onset Neonatal Group B Streptococcal Disease*. Green-Top Guideline No. 36. London: RCOG, November 2003.

Royal College of Obstetricians and Gynaecologists. *The Prevention of Early-Onset Neonatal Group B Streptococcal Disease in UK Obstetric Units*. London: RCOG, January 2007.

1.1.3 Uterine inversion

You are called to attend a collapsed patient on the labour ward.

A What is the estimated incidence of uterine inversion and what findings are associated with this condition? (4 marks)

B What are the symptoms and signs of uterine inversion? (5 marks)

C You diagnose uterine inversion in this case. What is your initial management? (6 marks)

D What are your options for replacement of the uterus? (5 marks)

Key words in the question

- Incidence, uterine inversion, findings, associated.
- Symptoms, signs.
- Uterine inversion, initial management.
- Options, replacement.

Essay plan

A

- 1/2000–1/6000.
- Short umbilical cord, morbidly adherent placenta, uterine anomalies.

B
- LAP, bleeding, shock.
- Non-palpable uterus, mass in vagina.

C
- Call help, resuscitate, immediate replacement uterus.
- Do not detach placenta.

D
- Replace +/− GA.
- O'Sullivan's.
- Surgery.

Suggested answer

A

The reported incidence of uterine inversion ranges from 1/2000 to 1/6000 (1).

Associated conditions include a short umbilical cord, a morbidly adherent placenta and uterine anomalies (3).

B

Signs and symptoms of uterine inversion include severe lower abdominal pain, bleeding, shock due to vagal stimulation, a non-palpable uterus or a dimpled fundus, and a mass in the vagina or outside the introitus (5).

C

For any collapsed patient the initial management is to call for help and to begin to resuscitate the patient (1).

Immediate replacement of the uterus should be attempted at the same time as beginning the resuscitation (1).

The patient should have two wide-bore cannulas inserted and blood taken for a full blood count, coagulation studies and cross-matching of four units of blood (1).

Fluid replacement should be given and observations for blood pressure, pulse and oxygen saturation should be commenced (2).

The placenta, if attached, should not be removed, as this may result in major bleeding (1).

D

There are a number of options available for replacement of the uterus. The first is manual replacement, preferably under general anaesthetic, as the uterus needs to be relaxed for replacement to succeed (1).

If this fails, then hydrostatic replacement (O'Sullivan's technique) can be used. Warm fluid, e.g. 0.9% saline, is infused into the posterior fornix, which stretches and relieves cervical constriction, allowing correction of the inversion (1).

Surgery is used if all other attempts fail. There are two techniques described. They are Huntingdon's procedure and Haultain's technique. Huntingdon's procedure involves the placement of Allis forceps in the dimple of the inverted uterus and using upward traction to replace the uterus. Haultain's technique involves making a vertical incision in the cervical ring posteriorly, which facilitates replacement of the uterus. The incision is then repaired (2).

Oxytocics should be administered after replacement of the uterus to ensure that the uterus remains contracted, to prevent recurrence (1).

Further reading

Wykes C. Uterine inversion. In: Grady K, Howell C, Cox C, eds. *Managing Obstetric Emergencies and Trauma. The MOET Course Manual* (2nd edition). London: RCOG Press, 2007: 239–44.

2 1.1.4 Cord prolapse

A Define cord prolapse and outline the difference between it and cord presentation. (2 marks)

B What is the incidence of cord prolapse and discuss the antenatal (non-procedural) risk factors associated with it? (8 marks)

C What procedures are associated with an increased risk of cord prolapse? (5 marks)

D What would you advise a paramedic in the community to do when faced with a cord prolapse prior to transfer to hospital? (5 marks)

Key words in the question

- Define, cord prolapse, outline, difference, cord presentation.
- Incidence, discuss, antenatal (non-procedural) risk factors.
- Procedures associated, cord prolapse.
- Advise, paramedic, community, cord prolapse, prior to transfer.

Essay plan

A

- Define occult and overt cord prolapse; cord prolapse through cervix, presentation between cervix and presenting part.

B

- Incidence ~0.5%; risk factors prevent application of presenting part to pelvis.

C

- Obstetric manipulations associated with cord prolapse.

D

- Manoeuvres to elevate fetus away from cord and transfer to hospital.

Suggested answer

A

Cord prolapse is defined as the descent of the umbilical cord through the cervix alongside (occult) or past the presenting part (overt) in the presence of ruptured membranes (1).

Cord presentation differs from cord prolapse in that it is the presence of the umbilical cord between the presenting part and the cervix instead of through the cervix. Cord presentation can occur with or without membrane rupture (1). *(with M. rupture = occult cord prolapse)*

B

The incidence of cord prolapse is approximately 0.5%. In breech presentation this rises to just over 1% (2).

Risk factors that may predispose to cord prolapse generally do so by preventing close application of the presenting part to the lower part of the uterus and/or pelvic brim. General factors include multiparity, low birthweight (less than 2.5 kg), prematurity (less than 37 weeks' gestation), fetal congenital anomalies, breech presentation, abnormal and unstable lie of the fetus, polyhydramnios, second twin, unengaged presenting part, and low-lying and abnormal placentation (6).

C

50% of cases of cord prolapse are preceded by an obstetric manipulation (1). The manipulation of the baby, as in external cephalic version for breech presentation and internal podalic version for the second twin, are both associated with cord prolapse (2). Manual rotation of the fetal head, artificial rupture of membranes and the placement of an intrauterine pressure catheter are also associated with cord prolapse (2).

D

I would advise a paramedic faced with a cord prolapse to get the woman to assume the knee–chest, face-down position (1). On getting to the ambulance this is best changed to left lateral position, as it is safer when moving (1). The patient should be transferred to the nearest consultant-led unit for delivery (1). If possible, the bladder should be filled naturally or via a Foley catheter to elevate the presenting part off the cord (1). The paramedic should be instructed to minimally handle the cord loops if outside the vagina, to prevent vasospasm (1).

Further reading

Royal College of Obstetricians and Gynaecologists. *Umbilical Cord Prolapse*. Green-Top Guideline No. 50. London: RCOG, April 2008.

1.1.5 Twin–twin transfusion

A 35-year-old woman attends the booking clinic at 12 weeks' gestation and ultrasound scan reveals a twin pregnancy.

A What are the important features of this pregnancy on ultrasound scan and why? (6 marks)

B How should her antenatal care be planned? (7 marks)

C What is twin-to-twin transfusion syndrome (TTTS) and how is it managed? (7 marks)

Key words in the question

- 12 weeks' gestation, twin pregnancy.
- Important features, ultrasound, why.
- Antenatal care.
- TTTS, managed.

Essay plan

A

- Number of fetuses and viability.
- Chorionicity.

B

- Anomaly scan.
- Regular scans.
- Antenatal steroids.
- Regular antenatal visits.

C

- Arteriovenous communication between placentae.
- Manage in fetal medicine unit.
- Regular antenatal checks with delivery after 34 weeks or earlier if needed.

Suggested answer

A

Important features on ultrasound scan are the number of fetuses and their viability (1). Determining the chorionicity at this stage is essential (1). In a dichorionic pregnancy there are two separate placental masses. If there is a single placenta, then the presence or absence of an intertwin membrane into the placental bed should be established. If present, a lambda sign suggests a dichorionic pregnancy and a 'T' sign suggests a monochorionic pregnancy (2).

Monochorionic pregnancies have a fourfold increase in the perinatal mortality compared with dichorionic twins. They also have more risk of preterm delivery and lower birthweight (2).

B

A twin pregnancy should be treated as a high-risk pregnancy and should be managed accordingly. A detailed anomaly scan should be arranged to pick up any structural defects (1).

Abdominal palpation for growth is of no value in twin pregnancies and therefore regular fetal biometry is recommended. In a monochorionic pregnancy, this should be arranged fortnightly from 22 weeks' gestation (1). In dichorionic twins, monthly scans are appropriate (1). If there are problems, more frequent visits and scans will be required.

Antenatal corticosteroids should be considered prophylactically in the third trimester, as there is a high risk of preterm delivery with twins (1).

Delivery should be planned in a unit with adequate neonatal facilities (1). The woman should have regular visits to the midwifery and obstetric clinics, as she is at higher risk of other obstetric complications, e.g. pre-eclampsia (1).

Should she remain undelivered, it is reasonable to offer induction of labour at 39–40 weeks, as there is a higher risk of antepartum stillbirth with twins (1).

C

TTTS occurs when unidirectional transfusion takes place from one fetus, acting as the donor, to the other fetus, acting as the recipient (1). This results from blood exchange in deep arteriovenous connections between the placentae in a monochorionic pregnancy (1). [This causes the donor twin to be small, with oligohydramnios, while the recipient twin becomes larger and develops polyhydramnios.]

Regular ultrasound is the main modality for monitoring TTTS (1). On diagnosis, referral should be made to a fetal medicine unit, where the connecting vessels may be obliterated by laser. Amniodrainage may be needed for the recipient twin (2). Antenatal steroids should be administered once viability has been attained (1).

Delivery by caesarean section should be considered once the patient reaches 34 weeks' gestation (1).

Further reading

Cameron A, Macara L, Brennand J, Milton P. *Fetal Medicine for the MRCOG and Beyond*. London: RCOG Press, 2002: 123–37.

1.1.6 Gestational diabetes

A primigravid woman at 28 weeks' gestation is referred from midwifery-led care with an ultrasound diagnosis of a macrosomic fetus but with no other abnormalities.

A What are the risk factors for gestational diabetes mellitus (GDM) and how is it diagnosed? (7 marks)

B If GDM is confirmed, how will her delivery be planned? (7 marks)

C What postnatal care and advice should she be given? (6 marks)

Key words in the question

- 28 weeks' gestation, macrosomic fetus.
- Risk factors, GDM.
- Delivery planned.
- Postnatal care, advice.

Essay plan

A

- BMI >30, previous history, large baby, family history, ethnic origin.
- Oral glucose tolerance test.

B

- Serial USS and estimate fetal weight.
- Hourly blood glucose measurement – may need intravenous insulin infusion.

C

- Stop all hypoglycaemic treatment.
- Early feed for baby.
- 6-week postnatal check for diabetes.
- Lifestyle advice.

Suggested answer

A

The risk factors for GDM are: a body mass index (BMI) $>30 \, \text{kg/m}^2$ (1); previous history of GDM (1); a baby with birthweight $>4.5 \, \text{kg}$ (1); and a family history of diabetes in a first-degree relative (1); GDM is more common in the Asian, Middle Eastern and Black Caribbean populations (1).

An oral glucose tolerance test should be organized between 24 and 28 weeks' gestation if any of these risk factors are present. This involves performing a fasting blood glucose measurement followed by an oral intake of 75 g of glucose. Diagnosis of GDM is confirmed if either fasting or 2-hour blood glucose levels are $>7.8 \, \text{mmol/l}$ (2).

B

Serial ultrasound scans will assess fetal well-being and estimate fetal weight near term (1). In the case of a macrosomic baby, the mother should be informed of the risks and benefits of vaginal birth versus caesarean section and an informed decision made (1). In view of the risks of shoulder dystocia and a 10-fold increase in the risk of Erb's palsy in a macrosomic fetus, a caesarean section is usually recommended (2).

An induction of labour can be offered after 38 completed weeks if the estimated fetal weight is $<4.5 \, \text{kg}$ (1).

During labour, hourly measurements of capillary blood glucose levels should be performed, with an attempt to maintain the level between 4 and 7 mmol/l (1).

If this is not achieved or the mother has been started on insulin during pregnancy, then her glycaemic control should be managed by an intravenous dextrose and insulin infusion in the form of a sliding scale (1).

C

Her hypoglycaemic treatment should be discontinued immediately after birth (1).

The baby should receive a feed, preferably be breast fed, within 30 minutes of birth and every two to three hours after that. Neonatal blood glucose levels should be monitored, as advised by the paediatricians (1).

She should be advised to have a fasting blood glucose measurement at 6 weeks after the birth and annually thereafter, as she has a 50% increased risk of developing type II diabetes mellitus within 10–15 years (2).

Lifestyle advice, such as weight control, diet and exercise, should be offered (1).

As she is at risk of GDM in future pregnancies, a glucose tolerance test should be performed early in her next pregnancy (1).

Further reading

Confidential Enquiry into Maternal and Child Health. *Pregnancy in Women with Type I and Type II Diabetes in 2002–03, England, Wales and Northern Ireland*. London: CEMACH, 2005.

Nelson-Piercy C. Diabetes. In: *Handbook of Obstetric Medicine* (3rd edition). London: Informa Healthcare, 2006: 82–99.

1.1.7 Non-immune hydrops

A 24-year-old woman who is 25 weeks' pregnant contacts her community midwife as her daughter has just been diagnosed with 'slapped cheek' syndrome. She is concerned about the potential effects of her daughter's illness on her pregnancy. The midwife contacts the hospital for advice.

A   What advice should the patient receive at this stage? (6 marks)

B   Two weeks later this woman's fetus develops non-immune hydrops (NIH). How should this be investigated? (9 marks)

C   Assuming the NIH is due to infection following her daughter's 'slapped cheek' syndrome, how should this be managed antenatally? (5 marks)

Key words in the question

- 25 weeks' pregnant, daughter, diagnosed, 'slapped cheek' syndrome, concerned, potential effects, pregnancy.
- Advice, at this stage.
- Fetus develops NIH, investigated.
- NIH, 'slapped cheek' syndrome, managed, antenatally.

Essay plan

A

- Reassurance for patient – not teratogenic but risk of NIH.
- Check for mother's B19 IgM and IgG status.
- Fetal surveillance.

B

- Likely parvovirus B19. Detailed history and maternal FBC, blood group and antibodies, Kleihauer, infection screen, autoantibodies, oral GTT.
- Detailed fetal ultrasound and fetal echocardiography.
- Fetal blood testing – cordocentesis.

C

- Mild – follow-up with ultrasound.
- Severe – intrauterine transfusion.

Suggested answer

A

The patient should be reassured that parvovirus B19 ('slapped cheek' syndrome) is not teratogenic and she can continue with her pregnancy (1). She should be advised to avoid contact with other pregnant women until she is proven to be immune or is non-infective (1). However, parvovirus B19 (PB19) is associated with non-immune hydrops (NIH), and some of these pregnancies result in fetal loss [up to 15%] (1). The greatest risk to the mother is when the infection occurs between 9 and 16 weeks. This pregnancy is 25 weeks so her risk of NIH is lower (1). She should be offered a blood test for PB19-specific IgM and IgG, which indicates recent infection and past infection, respectively. If only PB19-specific IgG is present, she can be reassured that her baby is not at risk of NIH (1). [50% of the adult population are immune.] If PB19-specific IgM is present, then she requires increased fetal surveillance with ultrasound scans to check for signs of fetal hydrops (1).

[Parvovirus B19 = erythema infectiosum = fifth disease is a mild influenza-type illness. The characteristic facial rash is called 'slapped cheek' syndrome. The rash appears approximately 16 days after infection and usually the patient is no longer infectious at this stage. The risk of a patient acquiring PB19 in pregnancy is approximately 1/400. In adults, the commonest symptom is arthralgia, especially in the hands and knees.]

B

Since NIH developed within a few weeks of this patient's daughter having 'slapped cheek' syndrome, the likely cause is fetal parvovirus B19 infection, and investigations should be focused with this in mind and the patient referred to a unit with fetomaternal expertise (1).

A detailed history should be obtained from the woman, particularly of recent infections, contacts or family history of metabolic disorders (1).

Maternal investigations should include full blood count, blood group and antibodies (to exclude immune causes), the Kleihauer test (for fetomaternal haemorrhage), and serology for parvovirus, toxoplasmosis, cytomegalovirus, rubella and syphilis (2).

An autoantibody screen for systemic lupus erythematosus, anti-Ro and La, and an oral glucose tolerance test should be performed (1).

A detailed fetal abnormality scan, including fetal echocardiography, should be performed. These tests help identify structural abnormalities such as cardiac defects and thoracic causes of hydrops, and may suggest chromosomal abnormality of the fetus (1). Amniotic fluid index, placental morphology and thickness and Doppler flow velocity studies should also be assessed (1). Cordocentesis should be performed after appropriate counselling. This permits diagnosis of chromosomal and metabolic disorders, and fetal infections, as specific IgM can be measured (2).

C

The management of NIH due to parvovirus B19 (PB19) will depend on its severity, as it is a potentially curable condition (1). A mild hydrops can often be managed conservatively with serial ultrasound scans, as spontaneous resolution may occur (1). However, failure of the hydrops to resolve or development of more severe hydrops necessitates invasive intervention. Fetal intrauterine blood transfusion is usually required, as PB19 may cause severe fetal anaemia (1). The patient needs to be warned about the risks of cordocentesis, which are increased in cases of NIH due to the precarious fetal condition (1). Frequently, one transfusion is sufficient and regular ultrasound monitoring confirms resolution (1).

Further reading

Cameron A, Macara L, Brennand J, Milton P. *Fetal Medicine for the MRCOG and Beyond*. London: RCOG Press, 2002: 87–99.

1.1.8 Thyroid disease

A woman attends the antenatal clinic at 20 weeks' gestation. Investigations show she has thyrotoxicosis due to Graves' disease.

A Identify three of the more discriminatory features of hyperthyroidism in pregnancy. (3 marks)

B How is thyrotoxicosis caused by Graves' disease diagnosed and what are the risks to this pregnancy? (8 marks)

C Outline your management of this woman's thyrotoxicosis. (7 marks)

D What are the indications for thyroidectomy in pregnancy? (2 marks)

Key words in the question

- 20 weeks' gestation, thyrotoxicosis, Graves' disease.
- Three, discriminatory features, hyperthyroidism, pregnancy.
- Thyrotoxicosis, diagnosed, risks, pregnancy.
- Management, thyrotoxicosis.
- Indications, thyroidectomy, pregnancy.

Essay plan

A

- Weight loss, tremor, tachycardia.

B

- Raised free T4, T3. Suppressed TSH. TSH receptor-stimulating antibodies.
- Well-controlled outcome usually good. Untreated risk IUGR, prematurity, perinatal death. Thyroid crisis with heart failure. Retrosternal goitre.

C

- Need endocrinologist.
- Anti-thyroid drugs, PTU preferred.
- TFTs and review monthly.
- Beta-blocker initially.

D

- Pressure symptoms, cancer, allergy to anti-thyroids.

Suggested answer

A

Three of the more discriminatory features of hyperthyroidism in pregnancy are weight loss, tremor and a persistent maternal tachycardia. (3) [Also lid lag and exophthalmos – this indicates thyroid disease at some time.]

B

Thyrotoxicosis is diagnosed by finding a raised free thyroxine (T4) or free tri-iodothyronine (T3) level (1). [Normal pregnant ranges for each trimester must be used.] Thyroid-stimulating hormone (TSH) is suppressed (1). Graves' disease is an autoimmune disorder caused by TSH receptor-stimulating antibodies. The presence of these antibodies in the blood confirms the diagnosis (1).

If this woman is well controlled on propylthiouracil (PTU), the maternal and fetal outcomes are usually good (1). However, if the thyrotoxicosis is untreated or poorly controlled, there is an increased risk of intrauterine growth retardation, premature labour and perinatal mortality (2). [Miscarriage is also increased.] At the time of delivery, poorly controlled thyrotoxicosis may lead to a thyroid crisis and heart failure (1). Very occasionally, a goitre may extend retrosternally, which may cause tracheal obstruction, rendering intubation difficult (1).

C

This patient's thyrotoxicosis should be managed in conjunction with an endocrinologist (1). The mainstay of treatment is anti-thyroid drugs, e.g. PTU and carbimazole (1). The aim is to render this woman euthyroid as rapidly as possible (1). PTU is preferable to carbimazole in this case because less of it crosses the placenta (1). She should be aggressively treated with high doses of PTU for four to six weeks. Following this the dose can usually be reduced (1). She should be reviewed monthly and have thyroid function tests (TFTs) checked. [Once stable, TFTs can be measured less frequently than monthly.] Often propranolol (a beta-blocker) is used in the early management of thyrotoxicosis to improve sympathetic symptoms, e.g. tachycardia and tremor (1). They can be discontinued once the woman's symptoms have improved (1).

D

The indications for thyroidectomy include pressure symptoms, e.g. dysphagia, a suspected thyroid cancer and allergy to PTU and carbimazole (2).

Further reading

Nelson-Piercy C. Thyroid and parathyroid disease. In: *Handbook of Obstetric Medicine* (3rd edition). London: Informa Healthcare, 2006: 100–15.

1.1.9 Obesity in pregnancy

A chronically morbidly obese patient undergoes emergency caesarean section (CS) at full cervical dilatation.

A What difficulties might the obstetrician encounter during CS? (5 marks)

B Describe possible postoperative complications and how you might reduce them. (11 marks)

C What pre-existing diseases might a patient who is chronically morbidly obese have at booking for antenatal care? (4 marks)

Key words in the question

- Grossly obese, emergency CS, full dilatation.
- Difficulties, encounter, CS.
- Postoperative complications, reduce.
- Pre-existing diseases, chronically morbidly obese.

Essay plan

A

- Difficult technically, LUS and uterine angle tear.
- Due to panniculus, haemostasis more difficult.
- CS takes longer.
- Pfannenstiel best.

B

- Morbidity higher.
- Wound infection.
- VTE.
- Chest infection.
- Higher risk of maternal death.

C

- DM, hypertension, IHD and PCOS.

Suggested answer

A

Her obesity is likely to result in the caesarean section (CS) being technically more difficult (1). The lower uterine segment may be more difficult to expose and if a uterine angle tear should occur, this is often more difficult to deal with than in a patient with a normal body mass index (BMI) (1). Due to the large panniculus, it may not be possible to exteriorize the uterus to facilitate suturing of the torn uterine angles and securing haemostasis (1). The duration of CS is prolonged in obese women, which means the surgeon must concentrate for longer (1). Despite these difficulties, a Pfannenstiel or low transverse incision is suitable for the vast majority of morbidly obese women, as a midline incision is associated with an increased incidence of wound dehiscence and chest infection (due to pain on inspiration) (1).

B

Postoperative morbidity is significantly higher after emergency surgery and in obese patients (1). Wound infection is more common due to the overhanging pannus (1). This risk may be reduced by meticulous attention to haemostasis, ligating larger blood vessels and applying diathermy to smaller bleeding points in the fat tissue. Furthermore, a fat suture to the adipose tissue reduces tension on the skin sutures and obliterates the dead space. An interrupted skin suture is probably best, in that if a small haematoma or localized collection occurs a few sutures may be removed to facilitate resolution. Careful abdominal wound toilet also helps reduce wound infection (3).

Venous thromboembolism is much higher in obese women (1). To reduce this risk, patients should be fitted preoperatively with thromboembolic stockings and continue wearing them for up to six weeks after surgery (1). Low-molecular-weight heparin should be given according to a protocol for obese patients (1).

Due to restriction in chest movement, chest infections are more common in obese patients postoperatively (1). Consideration should be given to pro-phylactic chest physiotherapy postoperatively (1).

Obesity is associated with an increased risk of maternal death (1). [In the most recent Confidential Enquiry (2003–5), more than 50% of mothers who died were overweight.]

C

A woman who is chronically morbidly obese may have pre-existing diabetes mellitus (1), hypertension (1), ischaemic heart disease (1) and/or polycystic ovarian syndrome (1).

Further reading

Irvine L, Shaw R. The impact of obesity on obstetric outcomes. *Current Obstetrics and Gynaecology* 2006; **16**: 242–6.

4

1.1.10 Cardiopulmonary arrest

You are the registrar on call for the labour ward and you are called to attend a collapsed patient in triage who was admitted at 34 weeks' ges-tation with a swollen left leg.

A What is your initial management of this situation? (3 marks)

B How would you diagnose a cardiopulmonary arrest? (4 marks)

C Assuming that this patient has had a cardiopulmonary arrest, describe how you would perform basic life support. (6 marks)

D How would you use an automated external defibrillator (AED) and what are the two shockable rhythms? (6 marks)

E What is the likely diagnosis? (1 mark)

Key words in the question

- Registrar, labour ward, collapsed patient, 34 weeks' gestation, swollen left leg.
- Initial management.
- Diagnose cardiopulmonary arrest.
- Basic life support.
- Automated external defibrillator (AED), two shockable rhythms.
- Likely diagnosis.

Essay plan

A

- Safe environment.
- Shake and shout.
- Call for help.

B

- Assess airway.
- Assess breathing.
- Check for carotid pulse.

C

- Left lateral tilt.
- 30 chest compressions to 2 ventilation breaths.

D

- Attach 2 adhesive pads and connect to machine.
- If shock advised make sure 'all clear'.
- Ventricular tachycardia and ventricular fibrillation.

E

- Pulmonary embolism.

Suggested answer

A

I would ensure the surrounding environment is safe before approaching the patient (1).

I would initiate a 'shake and shout' of the patient to establish if she is responding (1).

If there is no response, then, prior to initiating resuscitation, I would call out for help (1).

B

I would assess the airway. The mouth should be opened and checked for a foreign body, which should be removed if present. The head should be tilted back and the chin lifted. The jaw can be thrust forward if needed (1).

I would assess breathing by looking, listening and feeling for breath sounds. This should take no more than 10 seconds (1).

While doing this, the circulation can be checked by feeling for a carotid pulse (1).

If there is no breathing or circulation, then a cardiopulmonary arrest can be diagnosed (1).

C

The patient is pregnant and should be tilted between 15–30 degrees from the horizontal towards the left to minimize the effects of the gravid uterus on venous return (1).

Chest compressions should be initiated on the chest in the middle of the lower half of the sternum (1).

Compressions should be to a depth of 4–5 cm and at a rate of 100 beats per minute (2).

After 30 compressions 2 ventilation breaths should be given via a self-inflating bag (2).

D

The patient should be connected to the AED via two adhesive pads. The first pad is attached to the right of the sternum below the right clavicle. The other is attached in the left mid-axillary line, taking care to avoid the breast (2).

The pads are connected to the AED and the machine is switched on. The AED assesses the rhythm and advises when a shock is indicated (1).

If a shock is indicated, the operator must ensure that the resuscitation team stand well clear before the shock is initiated (1).

The two shockable rhythms are ventricular fibrillation and ventricular tachycardia (2).

E

The likely diagnosis is pulmonary embolism (1). [Swollen leg points to deep vein thrombosis, which may lead to pulmonary embolism.]

Further reading

Grady K, Prasad BGR, Howell C. Cardiopulmonary resuscitation in the nonpregnant and pregnant patient. In: Grady K, Howell C, Cox C, eds. *Managing Obstetric Emergencies and Trauma. The MOET Course Manual* (2nd edition). London: RCOG Press, 2007: 21–30.

1.1.11 Vaginal birth after caesarean section (VBAC)

A 32-year-old woman in her second pregnancy attends the antenatal clinic at 24 weeks' gestation to discuss the method of delivery for her current pregnancy. She had an emergency caesarean section for fetal distress at 6 cm last time.

A What are the contraindications to vaginal birth after caesarean section (VBAC) in general? (5 marks)
B Outline the risks and benefits of VBAC. (11 marks)
C What intrapartum support would you plan for this labour? (4 marks)

Key words in the question

- Second pregnancy, method of delivery, emergency caesarean section.
- Contraindications, vaginal birth.
- Risks, benefits.
- Intrapartum support.

Essay plan

- Previous uterine rupture, previous classical incision, >3 CS, J–incision.
- Compare risks and benefits of VBAC compared with elective C/S.
- Monitoring and precautions to be used in labour.

Suggested answer

A

Vaginal birth after caesarean section (VBAC) is contraindicated in women where there has been a previous uterine rupture. In this scenario, the risk of repeat rupture is unknown. VBAC is also contraindicated in those women who have had a previous high vertical classical caesarean section, where the risk of rupture can be as much as 9%. It is also not recommended in patients who have had three or more caesarean sections, although there are no reliable figures on risk. Women with an inverted T- or J-incision and women with a prior low vertical incision may have relative contraindications, with rupture rates of approximately 2% (4).

Although the evidence suggests that there is no statistically increased risk of rupture in those women with two previous caesarean sections compared with those with only one, there is an increased risk of hysterectomy and blood transfusion (1).

B

Risks
There is a risk of uterine rupture of up to 0.75% in women opting for a VBAC compared with virtually no risk in women opting for elective caesarean section (1).

Planned VBAC carries an increased risk of blood transfusion of approximately 1% compared with elective caesarean section (1).

There is also an increase of 1% in the risk of postpartum endometritis (1).

There is an increased risk of 2–3/10,000 of birth-related perinatal death compared with elective caesarean section. This is comparable to the risk for women having their first birth (1).

Planned VBAC carries an 8/10,000 risk (compared with 0 for elective caesarean section) of the baby developing hypoxic ischaemic encephalopathy (HIE). The long-term effect on the baby, however, remains unclear (1).

The chance of achieving a vaginal birth after a single caesarean section is approximately 75%, given an emergency caesarean section rate of 25% (1).

Benefits
VBAC reduces the chance that the baby will have respiratory problems after birth by up to half (2–3% from 3–4%) (1).

Repeat caesarean section increases the risk in subsequent delivery of placenta accreta, visceral injury to bladder, bowel or ureter, hysterectomy, admission to intensive care unit (ICU), blood transfusion and length of hospital stay (4).

C

VBAC should be undertaken in a suitably staffed and equipped labour ward, with continuous monitoring of the fetus and access to immediate caesarean delivery and neonatal resuscitation (1).

Women should be advised to have continuous electronic fetal monitoring from the onset of uterine contractions for the duration of the VBAC (1).

Continuous intrapartum care should allow for prompt identification and management of scar rupture by looking at the cardiotocography, observing for abdominal pain (particularly if it persists between contractions), scar tenderness, vaginal bleeding, maternal tachycardia, hypotension or shock, and loss of the station of the presenting part (2).

Further reading

Royal College of Obstetricians and Gynaecologists. *Birth After Previous Caesarean Birth*. Green-Top Guideline No. 45. London: RCOG, February 2007.

2   **1.1.12   Ovarian cysts in pregnancy**

A 34-year-old woman is seen in the antenatal clinic with an asymptomatic adnexal mass identified on ultrasound scan (USS) at 11 weeks' gestation.

A   Give four causes of an adnexal mass in pregnancy. (Assume the pregnancy is intrauterine.) (4 marks)

B   In what percentage of pregnancies are adnexal masses reported on USS? (1 mark)

C   Discuss the management of this case, assuming the adnexal mass was ovarian. (13 marks)

D   Is there a role for assessment of tumour markers in ovarian cysts in pregnancy? (2 marks)

Key words in the question

- Four, causes, adnexal mass, pregnancy.
- Percentage, pregnancies, adnexal masses, reported.
- Management, adnexal mass, ovarian.
- Role, tumour markers, ovarian cysts, pregnancy.

Essay plan

A

- Ovarian cysts, hydrosalpinx, paratubal cysts, fibroids.

B

- 5%.

C

- Depends on features.
- Majority resolve.
- USS 4 weeks.
- Reassure or surgery.

D

- Tumour markers CA125, serum AFP, βhCG.
- All elevated, limited use.

Suggested answer

A

Four causes of adnexal mass in pregnancy are ovarian cysts, hydrosalpinx, paratubal cysts and fibroids. [Ovarian cysts include simple, haemorrhagic, endometrioma, epithelial tumours, and germ cell tumours. Other, non-gynaecological causes include mesenteric cysts, diverticular disease and pelvic kidney.] (4)

B

Adnexal masses occur in up to 5% of all pregnant women. (1)

C

The management of this case depends on the size of the ovarian cyst, its appearance and whether the woman develops any symptoms (2). If the cyst is less than 5 cm in diameter and is simple in nature on ultrasound scan (USS), then further evaluation is not required unless pain develops (1). The majority of simple cysts resolve and the woman should be reassured of this (1). A simple cyst greater than 5 cm or any complex cyst needs further evaluation. This is usually via USS one month later to assess whether the cyst is enlarging (1). If the USS is inconclusive, then magnetic resonance imaging can be used to gain further information (1). If the cyst is not enlarging, then it should be re-examined six weeks postnatally (1). If there is a rapid increase in size or symptoms of pain, torsion or pressure develop, then surgery can be considered. If the cyst is simple, then fine-needle aspiration may be performed, although the patient needs to be aware that cysts recur in up to 50% of cases (1).

Surgery (via laparoscopy or laparotomy) can be performed to remove the cyst (1). If a laparoscopy is performed, then the Hasson (open) technique for entry into the abdomen should be employed, to minimize trauma to the pregnant uterus (1). The surgery should be performed after 14 weeks' gestation to minimize the risk of miscarriage due to damage to the corpus luteum (1). Care should be used to avoid intra-abdominal spillage of cyst contents (1). If there is any suspicion of malignancy, then a frozen section may be performed with subsequent oophorectomy and examination of the other ovary and subsequent biopsy if indicated (1).

D

The usual tumour markers in ovarian cancer – CA125, serum alpha-feto-protein (AFP) and beta-human chorionic gonadotrophin (βhCG) – are all elevated in pregnancy and therefore are of limited use (2).

Further reading

Spencer CP, Roberts PJ. Management of adnexal masses in pregnancy. *The Obstetrician and Gynaecologist* 2006; 8: 14–19.

1.1.13 Alcohol in pregnancy

A 36-year-old attending the antenatal booking clinic smells of alcohol. On questioning she admits to regular binge drinking (>5 drinks at one session) and a heavy alcohol intake for the past two years.

A What advice would you give this woman? (7 marks)

B Outline the potential risks to this pregnancy related to her alcohol intake. (9 marks)

C What are the diagnostic criteria for fetal alcohol syndrome (FAS)? (4 marks)

Key words in the question

- Booking clinic, alcohol, regular binge drinking, heavy alcohol intake, two years.
- Advice.
- Potential risks, pregnancy.
- Diagnostic criteria, FAS.

Essay plan

A

- Harm to fetus – binge drinking may be particularly harmful.
- Important to reduce intake.
- Counselling and detoxification programmes.
- Damage can occur throughout pregnancy.
- Enquire re other behaviours e.g. drug misuse.
- Treat with compassion.

B

- Increased risk of miscarriage, structural malformations, preterm delivery, IUGR, low birthweight, neurodevelopmental disorder, FAS, perinatal death, increased susceptibility to disease in adult life.

C

- Maternal exposure to alcohol.
- Characteristic facial anomalies.
- Growth restriction.
- Neurodevelopment abnormalities.

Suggested answer

A

This woman should be informed that heavy alcohol consumption and binge drinking in early pregnancy may be particularly harmful to her unborn baby (1).

She should be advised either to stop drinking or to reduce her intake to one or two units of alcohol once or twice a week (1).

Since alcohol-related damage can occur throughout pregnancy, the infant can benefit if the patient can be persuaded to reduce or stop drinking during pregnancy (1).

The patient may have other problems, such as drug misuse, poor nutrition and smoking, and it is important to try to identify these behaviours and offer advice (1).

She should be treated with compassion and respect, as failure to do so may result in her ceasing to attend for antenatal care (1).

She should be offered counselling and referral to a detoxification programme if necessary. Evidence suggests that interventions to reduce alcohol consumption in pregnancy are effective (2).

B

The risks to this pregnancy from heavy alcohol ingestion include an increased risk of miscarriage (1), aneuploidy (1), structural congenital abnormalities (1), intrauterine growth retardation (1), preterm delivery (1), perinatal death (1), developmental delay (1), fetal alcohol syndrome (FAS) (1) and susceptibility to disease in adult life (1).

C

The diagnostic criteria for FAS are confirmed maternal alcohol exposure (1), evidence of the characteristic facial anomalies, e.g. flat upper lip and flat mid-face (1), evidence of growth restriction, e.g. low birthweight for gestational age (1), evidence of neurodevelopmental abnormalities, e.g. microcephaly or agenesis of the corpus callosum, or decreased cranial size at birth or neurological hard or soft signs (1).

Further reading

Royal College of Obstetricians and Gynaecologists. *Alcohol Consumption and the Outcomes of Pregnancy*. RCOG Statement No. 5. London: RCOG, March 2006.

1.1.14 Preterm premature rupture of membranes

A 37-year-old primigravida with a pregnancy from in vitro fertilization and normal antenatal progress presents to the antenatal day unit (ANDU) at 26 weeks' gestation with a history suggestive of ruptured membranes.

A Outline your immediate management. (10 marks)

B Assuming rupture of membranes is confirmed, describe your subsequent management. (10 marks)

Key words in the question

- 37-year-old, primigravida, in vitro fertilization, 26 weeks' gestation, ruptured membranes.
- Immediate management.
- Subsequent management.

Essay plan

A

- Recognize likelihood of patient anxiety.
- Establish diagnosis.
- Assess maternal and fetal condition.
- Ascertain availability of neonatal facilities and cot.

B

- Expectant management.
- Prophylactic antibiotics and steroids.
- Regular monitoring of patient and fetus.
- Plan for delivery.

Suggested answer

A

This patient is likely to be very anxious, given her history of in vitro fertilization at the age of 37, and this should be acknowledged at the beginning of the consultation (1).

A history of fluid per vaginum and sterile speculum examination demonstrating pooling of fluid in the posterior fornix confirms the diagnosis. In uncertain cases, ultrasound is helpful if oligohydramnios is present (2).

Digital examination should be avoided, to reduce the risk of intrauterine infection (1).

If diagnosis of rupture of membranes (ROM) is confirmed, the patient should be admitted. If excluded, the patient may be discharged (1).

Useful investigations include white-cell count, high vaginal swab and temperature. Assessment of fetal heart rate and monitoring of uterine activity is performed using cardiotocography (2).

The availability of a neonatal cot and facilities must be discussed with the paediatricians. If unavailable, the patient should be given steroids, tocolysis prophylactically and transferred to another unit (2).

The diagnosis and plan of management are explained to the patient (1).

B

If the patient is not in labour, she is managed expectantly. Erythromycin (250 mg q.d.s. for 10 days) and steroids (e.g. intramuscular betamethasone 12 mg two doses 24 hours apart) are commenced (2).

If the patient starts contracting, tocolysis with atosiban or nifedipine is provided to permit the steroids to take effect. There is no proven benefit to using tocolysis beyond this time (1).

A senior paediatrician should counsel the patient regarding fetal outcomes at early gestations (1).

Serial ultrasounds for liquor volume and presentation weekly and growth every fortnight are arranged (1).

After 48–72 hours of observation, the patient may go home provided she is aware of symptoms and signs of chorioamnionitis. She should monitor her temperature twice a day and be followed up regularly in the ANDU (2).

Conservative management is continued until 34 weeks, and then induction of labour is offered if the presentation is cephalic, or caesarean section if breech (1).

Should any signs of chorioamnionitis develop (offensive vaginal discharge, fetal tachycardia and temperature), immediate delivery is undertaken (2).

Further reading

Royal College of Obstetricians and Gynaecologists. *Preterm Prelabour Rupture of Membranes*. Green-Top Guideline No. 44. London: RCOG, November 2006.

1.1.15 Consent to caesarean section

You are the registrar on the labour ward. You are asked to obtain Mrs Smith's consent for her elective caesarean section for breech presentation.

A Describe to Mrs Smith (in non-medical language) what the procedure involves. (7 marks)

B What are the alternatives to delivery by caesarean section for Mrs Smith and what are the risks? (8 marks)

C What are the serious risks of caesarean section you would discuss with Mrs Smith? (5 marks)

Key words in the question

- Consent, elective caesarean section, breech presentation.
- Describe, procedure, non-medical language.
- Alternatives to caesarean section, risks.
- Serious risks, caesarean section.

Essay plan

A

- Describe technique of CS as you would inform patient.

B

- ECV and vaginal breech delivery.

C

- Maternal, fetal, next pregnancy.

Suggested answer

A

The procedure will involve the delivery of the baby through the tummy, or abdomen (1).

Following the administration of an anaesthetic (usually spinal, which involves an injection in the back), a horizontal cut is made in the abdomen just above the pubic hairline (1).

The abdominal cavity is then opened and the bladder pushed out of the way (1).

A horizontal cut is made in the womb and the baby delivered (1).

The afterbirth is removed and the womb sewn up (1).

The abdomen is closed with stitches (1).

The whole procedure usually takes about 45 minutes (1).

B

The alternatives to caesarean section for Mrs Smith are external cephalic version (ECV) and planned vaginal breech delivery (2).

ECV is a safe option in breech presentation. There is an association between ECV and transient abnormal fetal heart rate patterns. Very occasionally, this may lead to fetal compromise and the need to deliver the baby immediately (1).

ECV is also associated with vaginal bleeding and placental abruption (2).

Planned vaginal breech delivery, when compared with caesarean section, is associated with an increase in perinatal and neonatal mortality and serious neonatal morbidity (1).

The Term Breech Trial (at two years) showed that there was no difference in outcome in the breech delivery and caesarean section groups for death and neurodevelopmental delay. The increase in death in the breech group was offset by an increase in the neurodevelopmental delay in the caesarean section group (2).

C

The serious risks for caesarean section can be divided into maternal risks, fetal risks and the risk in future pregnancies. Maternal risks include hysterectomy at 0.7%, the need for further surgery, and bladder and/or ureteric injury (0.3%), and death (1:12,000) (2).

Fetal risks are mainly lacerations, at approximately 2% (1).

In future pregnancies, the risk includes uterine rupture (0.4%) and an increased chance of placenta praevia and placenta accreta, at approximately 0.5% (2).

Further reading

Royal College of Obstetricians and Gynaecologists. *Caesarean Section.* Consent Advice No. 7. London: RCOG, May 2006.

Van Iddekinge B. Planned vaginal breech delivery: should this be the mode of choice? *The Obstetrician and Gynaecologist* 2007; 9: 171–6.

1.1.16 Renal disease in pregnancy

A primigravida attends booking clinic at eight weeks' gestation and gives a history of polycystic kidney disease.

A Outline the relevant management at this booking visit? (5 marks)

B She is diagnosed as having moderate renal impairment. What specific risks does she have during this pregnancy? (4 marks)

C How will you plan the management of her pregnancy? (5 marks)

D At 28 weeks' gestation she presents with fever, loin pain and rigors. A provisional diagnosis of acute pyelonephritis is made. How should this be managed? (6 marks)

Key words in the question

- Eight weeks' gestation, polycystic kidney disease.
- Management, booking visit.

- Moderate renal impairment, risks.
- Management, pregnancy.
- 28 weeks' gestation, acute pyelonephritis, managed.

Essay plan

A

- Establish baseline renal function.
- Start low-dose aspirin.

B

- Increased preterm labour and intrauterine growth restriction.
- Increased perinatal mortality.
- Hypertension.
- Pyelonephritis.

C

- Multidisciplinary approach.
- Regular assessment of renal function.
- Serial growth scans.
- 50% chance fetus will have polycystic kidneys.

D

- Aggressive antibiotic regime.
- Assess renal function.
- Avoid preterm labour.

Suggested answer

A

Any pre-existing history of renal impairment or family history of renal disease needs to be established (1). At this booking visit, note should be made of her blood pressure and the urine should be analysed for proteinuria (1). Her baseline renal function should be assessed by measuring of her urea and creatinine level, creatinine clearance, 24-hour protein excretion and a renal ultrasound (2). In view of the risks of hypertension in her pregnancy, she should be started on low-dose aspirin (1).

B

Approximately 50% of patients with moderate renal impairment will have a preterm delivery, with a third having intrauterine growth restriction (1). An increased perinatal mortality has also been recorded in these cases (1). These pregnancies are often complicated by hypertension, and if this is not adequately controlled the risks to the fetus and the maternal kidneys are increased. There is a possibility of accelerated decline in renal function in about a quarter of these patients (1). Patients with polycystic kidneys are at risk of acute pyelonephritis (1).

C

This patient should be managed in a multidisciplinary team comprising an obstetrician, an obstetric physician and a specialist midwife (1). Blood pressure and urinalysis should be closely monitored in the pregnancy (1). A regular creatinine clearance test will help to identify any deteriorating renal function. In such a case, referral to a nephrologist and early delivery may be recommended (1). Serial fetal growth scans should be arranged to identify developing growth restriction (1). Polycystic kidney disease is an autosomal dominant condition, and the woman should be made aware that there is a 50% chance of the baby being affected (1).

D

She needs to be admitted to hospital and a mid-stream urine specimen (MSU) sent for culture and sensitivity. Blood samples should be collected for full blood count and blood culture (1). Appropriate intravenous antibiotics (e.g. cephalosporins) should be started immediately and continued until the patient is apyrexial (1). The antibiotics may need to be altered based on the culture sensitivities. Oral antibiotics should then be continued for two weeks (1). Intravenous fluid may need to be administered in case of dehydration (1). Acute pyelonephritis may cause preterm labour and this will need to be dealt with by tocolysis and intramuscular steroid administration for fetal lung maturity (1). Renal function needs to be checked, as this can deteriorate in presence of sepsis (1).

Further reading

Nelson-Piercy C. Renal disease. In: *Handbook of Obstetric Medicine* (3rd edition). London: Informa Healthcare, 2006: 180–98.

1.1.17 Cardiac disease in pregnancy

A 22-year-old primigravida attends the booking clinic at 14 weeks' gestation. She has recently arrived in the UK from Pakistan and gives a history of rheumatic fever in childhood. On examination she is found to be mildly dyspnoeic.

A What is the most likely diagnosis? (1 mark)
B Outline appropriate antenatal management. (7 marks)
C How should her delivery be managed? (9 marks)
D How should she be managed in the puerperium? (3 marks)

Key words in the question

- 22-year-old primigravida, Pakistan, rheumatic fever, dyspnoeic.
- Likely diagnosis.
- Appropriate antenatal management.
- Delivery, managed.
- Managed, puerperium.

Essay plan

A

- Mitral stenosis.

B

- Cardiology assessment.
- Multidisciplinary management.
- Medical therapy, surgery — balloon valvuloplasty safe.
- Fetal assessment — serial USS as IUGR risk.

C

- Minimize additional load on cardiovascular system.
- Aim for vaginal delivery with assisted second stage. Effective analgesia.
- Avoid bolus doses of oxytocics.
- Antibiotic prophylaxis if assisted delivery/CS.
- Meticulous haemostasis essential.

D

- Monitor closely in immediate post-delivery period.
- Cardiology review.
- Contraception advice.

Suggested answer

A

The most likely diagnosis is rheumatic mitral stenosis (1).

B

This woman needs urgent cardiological assessment, including an echocardiogram (1). A multidisciplinary team consisting of an obstetrician, a cardiologist, a neonatologist and an anaesthetist should manage her (1). The frequency of antenatal visits and management will depend on the severity of the mitral stenosis and on whether it deteriorates during the pregnancy. Medical therapy aims to minimize volume overload. Pulmonary oedema should be treated with diuretics and beta-blockers used to slow the heart rate; cardioversion is appropriate if atrial fibrillation develops (2). Balloon mitral valvuloplasty may be required in cases refractory to medical treatment and is safe and effective in pregnancy (1).

Since there is a risk of intrauterine growth restriction, serial growth scans should be arranged in the third trimester (1). The patient should be advised to attend the hospital if she has signs of dyspnoea, persistent cough with pink frothy sputum (pulmonary oedema), or tachycardia, or feels unwell (1).

C

She should be delivered on a high-risk labour ward with appropriate midwifery, obstetric, and anaesthetic and cardiological backup support (1). The aim should be to minimize any additional load on her cardiovascular system during or after delivery (1). Spontaneous onset of labour with a vaginal delivery is preferable (1).

Induction of labour may be considered to optimize timing of delivery in relation to anticoagulation or because of deteriorating maternal cardiac function (1). Effective analgesia is recommended (as tachycardia is particularly dangerous in mitral stenosis) (1). Assisted vaginal delivery (ventouse or forceps) should be performed, as active maternal pushing is contraindicated (1).

The use of ergometrine (causes hypertension) or bolus of oxytocin (can cause hypotension) should be avoided and replaced by slow infusion of oxytocics (1).

Antibiotic prophylaxis is recommended for instrumental and surgical delivery, so this patient should be given antibiotics (1). With all surgical interventions, meticulous haemostasis is essential to avoid haemorrhage, as this increases the risk of cardiovascular instability (1).

D

This patient requires close monitoring for up to 72 hours after delivery while the main haemodynamic challenges settle. Multidisciplinary surveillance is maintained until the woman is fit for discharge (1). Multidisciplinary follow-up assessment is recommended at six weeks. Depending on the severity of her mitral stenosis, this patient may need regular cardiac outpatient follow-up or possibly surgery. (She arrived from Pakistan and was not known to have heart disease.) (1)

Contraception should be discussed with the patient so as to avoid an unplanned pregnancy. She requires a highly effective method such as Mirena or Implanon, as the consequences of contraceptive failure may be fatal if her cardiac disease deteriorates (1).

Further reading

Gelson E, Johnson M, Gatzoulis M, Uebing A. Cardiac disease in pregnancy, part 2: acquired heart disease. *The Obstetrician and Gynaecologist* 2007; **9**: 83–7.

Nelson-Piercy C. Heart disease. In: *Handbook of Obstetric Medicine* (3rd edition). London: Informa Healthcare, 2006: 22–39.

Steer PJ, Gatzoulis MA, Baker P, eds. *Heart Disease and Pregnancy.* Consensus Views Arising from the 51st Study Group. London: RCOG Press, November 2006.

1.1.18 Screening

A What are the principles of screening? (10 marks)

B What serum screening tests are available for Down syndrome? What are the detection rates, assuming a 5% false positive rate? (6 marks)

C Discuss the combined test for Down syndrome. (4 marks)

Key words in the question

- Principles of screening.
- Serum screening, Down syndrome, detection rates, 5% false positive.
- Discuss, combined test.

Essay plan

A

- WHO 10 principles for screening.

B

- Double, 59%; triple, 69%; quad, 76%.

C

- PAPP-A + βhCG + maternal age + NT − 85%.

Suggested answer

A

The principles of screening have been defined by the World Health Organiz-ation. There are 10 of these, as follows. The condition should be an important health problem (1). There should be treatment for the condition (1). Facilities and diagnosis for treatment of the condition should be available (1). There should be a latent stage of the disease (1). There should be a test or exam-ination for the condition (1). The test should be acceptable to the population (1). The natural history of the disease should be adequately understood (1). There should be an agreed policy on whom to treat (1). The total cost of finding a case should be economically balanced in relation to medical expen-diture as a whole (1). Case finding should be a continuous process, not just a 'once and for all' project (1).

B

The serum screening tests for Down syndrome: are the double test (alpha-fetoprotein and human chorionic gonadotrophin) (1), which has a detection rate of 59% (1); the triple test (double test plus unconjugated oestriol) (1), with a detection rate of 69% (1); and the quadruple test (triple test plus inhibin A) (1), which has a pick-up rate of 76% (1).

C

The combined test for Down syndrome is a combination of blood tests, maternal age and an ultrasound scan (1). The blood tests performed are pregnancy-associated plasma protein A (PAPP-A) and free beta-human chor-ionic gonadotrophin (1). The ultrasound determines fetal nuchal translucency, which is a measure of the fluid-filled space at the back of the fetal neck (1). The test is performed between 10 and 14 weeks' gestation and has a detection rate of 85% for a 5% false positive rate (1).

Further reading

Wilson JMG, Junger G. Principles and practice of screening for disease. *WHO Chronicle* 1968; **22**(11): 473.

www.screeningservices.org.uk/asw. This is the Antenatal Screening Wales website, which contains information on screening for Down syn-drome and the detection rate.

1.1.19 Blood transfusion in obstetrics

A How may the risk of blood transfusion be reduced in the obstetric population? (8 marks)

B Outline four risks of blood transfusion. (4 marks)

C Discuss four blood components that may be required in the treatment of massive obstetric haemorrhage and describe in what clinical situation they may be used. (8 marks)

Key words in the question

- Risk, blood transfusion, reduced.
- Four risks.
- Blood components, treatment, massive obstetric haemorrhage, clinical situation.

Essay plan

A

- Antenatal – oral and parenteral iron, rHuEPO.
- Delivery – active management of 3rd stage, anticoagulants, high risk of haemorrhage, advise hospital delivery.

B

- Mismatched blood products, infection, isoimmunization, TRALI.

C

- Red cells, FFP, cryoprecipitate, platelets.

Suggested answer

A

The risk of blood transfusion in pregnancy can be reduced by treating anaemia aggressively. If the antenatal Hb < 10.5 g/dl and investigations reveal iron deficiency anaemia, then oral iron should be prescribed (1).

If oral iron is unsuccessful at raising Hb levels, then parenteral iron is administered (1). Parenteral iron infusion results in a faster response than oral therapy but is more expensive (1). In specialist cases, e.g. a severely anaemic Jehovah's Witness unresponsive to parenteral iron, recombinant human erythropoietin (rHuEPO) may be considered (1). [The RCOG recommends this treatment only in the context of a clinical controlled trial; however, rHuEPO has been safely used antenatally and postpartum without adverse effects on mother or baby.]

The aim is to enter labour with an Hb level >10.5 g/dl so the patient has some reserve. At delivery, blood loss should be minimized to reduce the risk of the woman requiring a transfusion (1). Active management of the third stage of labour using oxytocics is effective at reducing blood loss (1). If the woman is on anticoagulants, optimal management will minimize blood loss (1). Should the patient be at a high risk of haemorrhage during labour, e.g. placenta praevia or a grand multiparous woman, she should be strongly advised to deliver in hospital (1).

B

The commonest risk of blood transfusion is transfusion of mismatched blood products (human error) (1). Other risks include transfusion-related infection (1), e.g. bacterial (Gram-negative with RBC and Gram-positive with platelets), viral (hepatitis B or C, HIV) or prion (e.g. variant Creutzfeldt–Jakob disease); immune sensitization (1) (e.g. Rh D antigen); and transfusion-related acute lung injury (TRALI) (1).

C

Four blood components useful in massive obstetric haemorrhage include red blood cells (RBCs) (1), fresh frozen plasma (FFP) (1), cryoprecipitate (1) and platelets (PLTs) (1).

RBCs are given when severe active haemorrhage is ongoing. Provided there are no irregular antibodies, group-specific compatible blood can be made available within 10 minutes (plus transport time). If irregular antibodies are present, cross-matching may be significantly delayed. In emergency situations O Rh D-negative red cells can be given (1).

FFP contains coagulation factors and cryoprecipitate is rich in fibrinogen. They are very useful in cases where disseminated intravascular coagulation (DIC) is present, e.g. severe PET (pre-eclamptic toxaemia), placental abruption or amniotic fluid embolism. They should be given as advised by a haematologist, who is guided by coagulation screens, full blood counts and the clinical situation (2).

The platelet count should be kept above $50 \times 10^9/l$ if possible. Platelet transfusion is seldom required. However, when needed it is prescribed on the advice of a haematologist (1).

Further reading

Maxwell MJ, Wilson MJA. Complications of blood transfusion. *Continuing Education in Anaesthesia, Critical Care and Pain* 2006; **6**: 225–9.
Royal College of Obstetricians and Gynaecologists. *Blood Transfusion in Obstetrics*. Green-Top Guideline No. 47. London: RCOG, December 2007.

1.1.20 Fetus small for gestational age

A primigravid patient is referred by her midwife to the antenatal assessment unit at 32 weeks' gestation with reduced fetal movements and a symphyseal–fundal height of 26 cm. An ultrasound scan suggests a fetus small for gestational age (SGA).

A What are the causes of a fetus being small for gestational age (SGA)? (7 marks)

B Outline appropriate antenatal care for the rest of this pregnancy. (8 marks)

C Identify the potential short- and long-term sequelae of a SGA fetus. (5 marks)

Key words in the question

- Primigravid, 32 weeks' gestation, reduced fetal movements, symphyseal–fundal height, 26 cm, ultrasound, SGA.
- Causes, SGA.
- Antenatal care.
- Potential short- and long-term sequelae, SGA fetus.

Essay plan

A

- Constitutional – the majority.
- Pathological – chromosome, congenital infection, structural abnormalities, teratogens.
- Unexplained – 'uteroplacental insufficiency'.

B

- Distinguish normal small from pathologically small.
- AFI, UAD, CTG useful.
- Consider karyotyping $+/-$ viral studies.

C

- Immediate and short-term sequelae.
- Effects in adulthood.

Suggested answer

A

The majority (about 60%) of fetuses small for gestational age (SGA) are constitutionally small; i.e. they are statistically small for their gestational age. They have grown at a constant velocity and are healthy (1).

Pathological causes of SGA babies include chromosomal abnormalities, e.g. trisomy 21, 18 and 13 (1); congenital infection with rubella, cytomegalovirus or toxoplasmosis (1); fetal structural abnormalities such as achondroplasia or gastroschisis (1); or first-trimester exposure to teratogens, e.g. excess alcohol or warfarin (1). Severe maternal systemic illness or malnutrition, heavy smoking or pregnancy-related conditions such as pre-eclampsia are associated with growth restriction in utero and may lead to SGA (1).

Abnormal uteroplacental development caused by failure of the second wave of trophoblastic invasion and failure of villous development leads to reduced flow of blood into the placental bed and limits the area available for uptake of gas and nutrients, resulting in fetal growth restriction. These cases of 'unexplained' growth retardation are attributed to 'uteroplacental insufficiency' (1).

B

One important (but often difficult) aim of further antenatal care is to distinguish the constitutionally small but healthy fetus from one that is pathologically small (1). Since the baby is small for gestational age, it would commonly have an abdominal circumference of <10th centile for 32 weeks' gestation. Ultrasound parameters such as amniotic fluid volume, umbilical artery Doppler studies and cardiotocography (CTG) would help assess this fetus further (1). If the scan suggests a structural abnormality is present with a normal liquor volume (LV) and umbilical artery Doppler (UAD), there is a substantial risk of chromosomal abnormality, and fetal karyotyping with appropriate counselling should be discussed (1). If the ultrasound scan reveals normal LV and normal UAD and no fetal anomaly, the small fetus is likely to be a 'normal small baby' (1). Outpatient management is safe and the patient should be monitored every two weeks with a scan and Doppler study (1). If the abdominal circumference and estimated fetal weight decrease further and

LV and UAD remain normal, karyotyping and viral studies may be considered (1). If there is reduced LV, absent or reversed end diastolic flow in the umbilical artery, then admission to hospital, intensive monitoring with CTG and daily LV, administration of steroids and early delivery are appropriate (2).

C

Constitutionally small fetuses born near term do not have any significant morbidity (1). However, SGA fetuses with growth restriction have an increased risk of stillbirth, intrapartum hypoxia, neonatal complications and impaired neurodevelopment (2).

In the adult life they have an increased tendency to develop hypertension, cardiovascular disease and type II diabetes (2).

Further reading

Cameron A, Macara L, Brennand J, Milton P. Intrauterine growth restriction. In: *Fetal Medicine for the MRCOG and Beyond*. London: RCOG Press, 2002: 109–22.

Royal College of Obstetricians and Gynaecologists. *The Investigation and Management of the Small-for-Gestational-Age Fetus*. Green-Top Guideline No. 31. London: RCOG, November 2002.

1.1.21 Genital herpes

A primigravida presents to the antenatal clinic at 36 weeks' gestation with a primary episode of genital herpes (GH).

A Justify your management. (10 marks)

B Another patient attends your antenatal clinic later the same day at term with a recurrent episode of genital herpes. Outline appropriate management. (7 marks)

C How may genital herpes infection in pregnancy be reduced? (2 marks)

D How may postnatal transmission of the herpes simplex virus (HSV) to the neonate be prevented? (1 mark)

Key words in the question

- 36 weeks' gestation, primary episode, GH.
- Justify, management.
- Recurrent, GH, management.
- Postnatal, HSV, neonate, prevented.

Essay plan

A

- Refer GUM, aciclovir, risks/benefits, HSV blood test, screen for other STIs.
- Offer CS. If declines CS, avoid invasive procedures.

B

- Most episodes short-lived. Antiviral treatment not required. Saline baths and analgesia.
- Risk neonatal herpes very small and CS not indicated.
- If membranes rupture, expedite delivery, avoid invasive procedures.
- Inform neonatologist.

C

- Use condoms, abstain, avoid orogenital contact with infected partner.

D

- Keep baby away from persons with active HSV infection.

Suggested answer

A

Once the patient has had her antenatal check she should be referred to the genitourinary medicine clinic (1). She should be prescribed aciclovir [200 mg five times daily for five days] and have a blood test for herpes simplex virus (HSV) antibody testing. Antibody testing can help distinguish between primary and recurrent infection. This is important, as recurrent genital herpes (GH) infection is associated with a very low risk of neonatal herpes (2).

The patient should be informed of the potential risks and benefits of aciclovir, as it is not licensed for use in pregnancy (1). Aciclovir reduces the severity and duration of symptoms and decreases viral shedding (1). The patient should be screened for other sexually transmitted infections (1).

Since the woman has a primary infection of GH and is within 6 weeks of delivery, she should be offered a caesarean section (CS). The purpose of the CS is to reduce exposure of the fetus to HSV in the maternal genital secretions (2). If the patient declines a CS, it is important to avoid rupture of membranes and invasive procedures in labour, such as fetal scalp electrode insertion or fetal blood sampling (1). The neonatologist should be informed and intravenous aciclovir considered for the patient (to reduce viraemia) and neonate (1).

B

This patient should be informed that most recurrent episodes are short-lived and resolve within 7–10 days (1). Antiviral treatment and cultures of lesions (to predict viral shedding) are not usually required (1). Supportive treatment with saline bathing and simple analgesia is appropriate (1). She should be informed that the risk of her baby having neonatal herpes is very small and that CS is not indicated (2). If rupture of membranes occurs, delivery should be expedited by the most appropriate method, e.g. intravenous oxytocin; or, if the cervix is very unfavourable, CS can be considered (1). Invasive procedures, e.g. insertion of fetal scalp electrode and fetal blood sampling, should be avoided. The neonatologist should be aware that the baby's mother has recurrent GH (1).

C

If the woman has no previous history of GH, she can reduce her risk of acquiring GH in pregnancy by using condoms or even abstaining from sexual intercourse (1).

She may also reduce her risk by avoiding orogenital contact with her partner if he has orolabial herpes (cold sores) (1).

D

To prevent postnatal HSV transmission, the mother must ensure she keeps her newborn away from any persons with active HSV infection, e.g. herpes labialis or herpetic whitlow [infection of the finger] (1).

Further reading

Royal College of Obstetricians and Gynaecologists. *Management of Genital Herpes in Pregnancy*. Green-Top Guideline No. 30. London: RCOG, September 2007.

1.1.22 Massive obstetric haemorrhage

A Define massive obstetric haemorrhage and state what the difficulty is in clinical practice with this definition. (2 marks)

B Apart from uterine atony, give two other major causes of obstetric haemorrhage. (2 marks)

C How do you define shock and what are the maternal signs of it? (5 marks)

D How would you treat a woman having an atonic postpartum haemorrhage (PPH), following active management of the third stage? (11 marks)

Key words in the question

- Define, massive obstetric haemorrhage, difficulty, definition.
- Apart from atony, two, causes.
- Shock, maternal signs.
- Treat, atonic PPH, active management, third stage.

Essay plan

A

- 1500+ ml, difficult to estimate loss.

B

- Placenta praevia, abruption.

C

- Inadequate tissue perfusion, tachycardia, BP, poor perfusion, confusion.

D

- Resuscitate patient, IV access, medical treatments, tamponade, surgery, radiology.

Suggested answer

A

Massive obstetric haemorrhage is defined as the loss of more than 1500 ml of blood either antepartum or postpartum (1). Problems arise clinically with the definition because the volume of blood loss is difficult to estimate accurately (1).

B

Apart from uterine atony, two other major causes of obstetric haemorrhage are placenta praevia and placental abruption (2). [Other causes include genital tract trauma, uterine rupture, uterine inversion, fibroids and retained placenta.]

C

Shock is defined as inadequate tissue perfusion, which can lead to imminent cell death (1). The maternal signs of shock include tachycardia, hypotension, tachypnoea, poor peripheral perfusion, confusion, oliguria and unexplained metabolic acidosis (4).

D

Assuming active management of the third stage and the use of syntocinon have already been performed, the first step is to call for help and begin resuscitation of the patient. At the same time, a contraction of the uterus can be rubbed up (1). If not already present, the insertion of two wide-bore cannulas is essential, and blood should be taken for full blood count and cross-matching of four units. Intravenous fluid replacement is commenced (1).

Once the cannulas are in place, then a further bolus of syntocinon 10 IU can be given. Ergometrine 0.5 mg can also be considered, as the effects are longer lasting than syntocinon (1). An infusion of syntocinon may be used to maintain a contraction [40 units in 500 ml 0.9% saline over 4 hours] (1). If this is unsuccessful, then prostaglandins may be considered. Carboprost [prostaglandin $F_{2\alpha}$ – $PGF_{2\alpha}$, 250 µg repeated every 15 minutes to a maximum of 2 g, has been successfully used following failure of conventional treatment. Misoprostol [800 µg rectally] is also effective (2). If this fails to control the bleeding, then the genital tract and uterus should be explored to exclude trauma and retained tissue (1). If this is negative, then uterine tamponade can be performed. This can be done by packing or by the utilization of a hydro-static balloon, such as a Rusch® balloon (1). Other options include laparotomy and surgical procedures such as arterial ligation of the uterine or internal iliac artery, the insertion of a B-lynch suture and, if all else fails, a hysterectomy (2). Some hospitals have access to interventional radiology, and in these units arterial embolization may be considered (1).

Further reading

Howell C, Irani S. Massive obstetric haemorrhage. In: Grady K, Howell C, Cox C, eds. *Managing Obstetric Emergencies and Trauma. The MOET Course Manual* (2nd edition). London: RCOG, 2007: 171–94.

1.1.23 Sickle cell disease in pregnancy

A 28-year-old woman with sickle cell disease attends your clinic, as she plans to start a family.

A What preconceptual evaluation is important? (5 marks)

B Outline the risks of sickle cell disease in pregnancy. (6 marks)

C How should her antenatal care be managed? (9 marks)

Key words in the question

- 28-year-old woman, sickle cell disease.
- Preconceptual evaluation, important.
- Outline, risks, sickle cell, pregnancy.
- Antenatal care, managed.

Essay plan

A

- Frequency of sickling, previous blood transfusions.
- Baseline end organ status.
- Antibiotic prophylaxis, vaccinations, folic acid.
- Partner screening.

B

- Fetal risks.
- Maternal risks.
- Sickle cell crisis.

C

- Multidisciplinary management. Folic acid, penicillin, vaccinations.
- Avoid 'triggers' of sickling, seek urgent medical help if suspect crisis.
- Blood and exchange transfusions – expert advice required.
- Baseline bloods.
- Every visit haemoglobin and MSU.
- Serial USS – risk IUGR – Dopplers.

Suggested answer

A

It is important to ascertain the frequency of sickling crises and any previous blood transfusions she may have had (1). Her cardiac (for heart failure), renal (for nephropathy) and lung function (for pulmonary hypertension) should be assessed for end organ damage, so she should be referred to a physician for this. Pregnancy is contraindicated if she has pulmonary hypertension, as maternal mortality approaches 50% (1). She should be advised to continue her antibiotic prophylaxis and to ensure she keeps up to date with immunizations [hepatitis B and pneumococcal] (1). Folic acid should be increased to 5 mg daily (1). Her partner should be screened for sickle cell disease or trait in order to give her an accurate estimate of the risk of having an affected child (1).

B

Complications of sickle cell disease are more common in pregnancy. There is an increased risk of miscarriage, intrauterine growth restriction, premature labour and fetal distress, and perinatal mortality is four to six times higher (2). Maternal risks include thromboembolism, pre-eclampsia and infections, particularly of the urinary tract and chest (pneumonia), and puerperal sepsis (2). Up to 35% of pregnancies are complicated by sickle crisis (1). Early, aggressive antenatal care has improved perinatal outcome and reduced maternal mortality to less than 1% (1).

C

Her antenatal care should be managed by a multidisciplinary team consisting of a haematologist, an anaesthetist and an obstetrician with an interest in maternal medicine (1). She should be advised to take folic acid supplementation at 5 mg/day, and it is important to confirm she is taking penicillin V 250 mg b.d. (as hyposplenism is common) and that she is up to date with hepatitis B and pneumococcal vaccines (1). The maternal and fetal risks should be explained and the need for close monitoring during pregnancy emphasized (1). She should be encouraged to avoid dehydration and cold environments, as either may trigger a sickling crisis. If she suspects infection or an impending crisis, she should seek medical help urgently (1). Blood transfusion may be required, e.g. for severe anaemia, and exchange transfusion if the patient is volume replete. Exchange transfusion is controversial in pregnancy, so expert haematological advice is essential (1).

Accurate dating using ultrasound is important, as sickle cell patients have an increased risk of intrauterine growth restriction (IUGR) and may need preterm delivery (1). Baseline full blood and reticulocyte count, serum ferritin, and liver and renal function tests are obtained. Iron supplementation should be given only if indicated (1).

Antenatal review is advisable every two to four weeks in the first and second trimester, with close liaison with a haematologist and haemoglobinopathy nurse specialist. As well as routine antenatal care, her haemoglobin and mid-stream urine should be checked at each visit (1). Serial growth scans should be performed in the third trimester, and if IUGR develops umbilical artery Doppler velocimetry and liquor volume measurements are recommended (1).

[Sickling crisis is treated using adequate analgesia, rehydration and antibiotics if infection is suspected. Aim for vaginal delivery – caesarean section is performed for obstetric indications only and regional anaesthetic is indicated to avoid desaturation precipitating a sickle crisis.]

Further reading

Nelson-Piercy C. Haematological problems. In: *Handbook of Obstetric Medicine* (3rd edition). London: Informa Healthcare, 2006: 254–7.

Ntim EO, Cottee C, Bewley S, Anionwu E. Sickle cell disease in pregnancy. *Current Obstetrics and Gynaecology* 2006; **16**: 353–60.

1.1.24 Thromboprophylaxis

A 27-year-old woman attends the antenatal booking clinic at 10 weeks' gestation. She gives a history of having had a deep vein thrombosis (DVT) when she returned from a holiday in Thailand.

A If she has no other risk factors, what counselling would you give her regarding thromboprophylaxis? (5 marks)

B Discuss pre-existing risk factors for venous thromboembolism in pregnancy. (8 marks)

C Under what other circumstances should antenatal thromboprophylaxis be considered? (7 marks)

Key words in the question

- 10 weeks' gestation, DVT.
- No other risk factors, advice, thromboprophylaxis.
- Risk factors, venous thromboembolism, pregnancy.
- Antenatal thromboprophylaxis.

Essay plan

A

- Avoid dehydration.
- Anticoagulate if immobile and in puerperium.
- Commence ASAP postpartum – caution with haemorrhage and epidural.

B

- Pregnancy, previous VTE, congenital and acquired thrombophilias, age, obesity, high parity, varicose veins.

C

- Previous recurrent VTE, previous VTE + family history, previous VTE + thrombophilia, thrombophilia + one additional risk factor, specific asymptomatic thrombophilias, previous VTE + antiphospholipid syndrome, three persisting risk factors.

Suggested answer

A

She should be advised to avoid dehydration and maintain an adequate fluid intake (1). If she has a period of immobility, she will require anticoagulation and anti-thrombotic stockings (1). She will need thromboprophylaxis for six weeks postnatally (1) with low-molecular-weight heparin or warfarin, as both are safe with breast-feeding (1). Thromboprophylaxis should be commenced as soon as possible postpartum, assuming there has been no haemorrhage. If she has an epidural catheter, the anticoagulant should be withheld until it has been removed (1).

B

Pregnancy itself is a risk factor for venous thromboembolism (VTE) (10-fold) because it is a hypercoaguable state (1). Pre-existing risk factors include previous VTE (1) and congenital thrombophilia states such as factor V Leiden, and protein C and S deficiency (1). Acquired thrombophilia states include antiphospholipid syndrome (1) [lupus anticoagulant and anticardiolipin antibodies]. Other pre-existing factors are age over 35 years (1), obesity (BMI >30 kg/m^2) (1), parity of four or more (1) and the presence of gross varicose veins (1). [Rarer risk factors are paraplegia, sickle cell disease, inflammatory disorders and myeloproliferative disorders.]

[New-onset and transient risk factors include surgical procedures performed in pregnancy, hyperemesis and dehydration, severe infection, pre-eclampsia, long-haul travel and immobility (greater than four days' bed rest).]

C

Women should be offered antenatal thromboprophylaxis if they have had a previous recurrent VTE (1) or a previous VTE and a family history of VTE in a first-degree relative (1). Patients with a previous VTE and an inherited thrombophilia should also be offered antenatal thromboprophylaxis (1). If a woman has an inherited thrombophilia but not a previous VTE, she should be offered antenatal prophylaxis if she has an additional risk factor (obesity, parity more than four, etc.) (1). However, if the asymptomatic thrombophilia is antithrombin deficiency, combined defects, homozygous factor V Leiden or prothrombin gene defect, the woman requires antenatal thromboprophylaxis (without the presence of any additional risk factors) (1). Patients with anti-phospholipid syndrome and a previous VTE should receive antenatal thromboprophylaxis (1). Women with three or more persisting risk factors should be considered for thromboprophylaxis antenatally (1) [varicose veins, parity more than four, obesity, age >35 years, antiphospholipid syndrome].

Further reading

Royal College of Obstetricians and Gynaecologists. *Thromboprophylaxis During Pregnancy, Labour and After Vaginal Delivery.* Green-Top Guideline No. 37. London: RCOG, January 2004.

1.1.25 Symphysis pubis diastasis

A patient at 34 weeks' gestation comes to see you in the antenatal clinic complaining of symptoms suggestive of symphysis pubis diastasis.

A What is the aetiology of this condition? (5 marks)
B What is the usual clinical presentation? (3 marks)
C What are the clinical signs and how is the diagnosis confirmed? (4 marks)
D What are the management options? (5 marks)
E How would you plan delivery of the baby? (3 marks)

Key words in the question

- 34 weeks' gestation, symphysis pubis diastasis.
- Aetiology.

- Clinical presentation.
- Signs, diagnosis confirmed.
- Management options.
- Plan delivery.

Essay plan

A

- Hormones, metabolic, trauma, poor posture and exercise.

B

- Pain and radiation, gait.

C

- Pain, gait, USS.

D

- Walking stick, belt, physiotherapy, analgesia, alternative therapies.

E

- Vaginal delivery, IOL if pain severe, no caesarean section.

Suggested answer

A

The aetiology of symphysis pubis diastasis (SPD) includes hormonal factors. Although this exact link has not been with a specific hormone, the link with hormonal factors appears undisputed. Increased relaxin, progesterone and oestrogen levels have all been implicated (1).

Metabolic factors, including decreased calcium and decreased vitamin D, have also been implicated (1).

The trauma of previous parturition and arthritis of pubic symphysis may have a role too (1).

Poor posture, lack of exercise and undertaking strenuous exercise in pregnancy are also thought to contribute (1).

General factors include age, weight gain and multiparity (1).

B

The classic symptoms of SPD include pain, which is localized to the pubis symphysis and described as shooting, burning, grinding and clicking (1).

This pain may radiate to the lower abdomen, groin and thigh (1).

It can be associated with difficulty in walking, climbing stairs and any weight-bearing activity (1).

C

The commonest clinical signs are tenderness over the sacroiliac joints and the symphysis pubis, with hip movement reduced due to pain. A waddling gait may also be present (2).

Imaging is the only way to confirm diastasis and ultrasound has been shown to be safe, but there has been no correlation shown between the size of the symphyseal gap and the severity of the symptoms (2).

D

The management options available to the patient include aids to stability such as walking sticks (1), a pelvic support with a trochanteric belt (1), specialist obstetric physiotherapy (1) and regular analgesia in the form of paracetamol and codeine-based preparations (1). Alternative therapies have been reported to be of benefit, including transcutaneous electrical nerve stimulation, ice and massage (1).

E

Spontaneous vaginal delivery is recommended in women with SPD (1).

Induction of labour may be offered to those women in extreme pain but only after the risks and benefits have been fully discussed with the woman (1).

There is no evidence to show that caesarean section is beneficial to women with SPD (1).

Further reading

Jain S, Eedarapalli P, Jamjute P, Sawdy R. Symphysis pubis dysfunction: a practical approach to management. *The Obstetrician and Gynaecologist* 2006; 8: 153–8.

1.1.26 Confidential enquiry into maternal and child health

The most recent report from the Confidential Enquiry into Maternal and Child Health (CEMACH), that for 2003–5, was published in December 2007.

A Outline three differences from previous reports. (3 marks)

B Discuss four objectives of the report. (4 marks)

C Define direct, indirect, coincidental and late deaths. Which type of death was the highest for this triennium? (5 marks)

D What were the commonest causes of direct and indirect death in this report? (2 marks)

E The maternal mortality rate has not declined since the mid-1980s. What factors have contributed to this lack of decline in deaths? (6 marks)

Key words in the question

- CEMACH.
- Three differences.
- Four objectives.
- Define direct, indirect, coincidental, late.
- Commonest.
- Maternal mortality, lack of decline.

Essay plan

A

- New title.
- 10 recommendations.
- Chapter on 'near misses'.

B

- Assess main causes, substandard care.
- Improve care of women.
- Recommendations for service provision.
- Audit, research.

C

- Definitions.

D

- Thromboembolism and cardiac disease.

E

- Maternal age, migrant mums, multiple births, health and lifestyle, lack of clinical skills, including resuscitation.

Suggested answer

A

Three differences from previous reports are: the name has changed from 'Why Mothers Die' to 'Saving Mothers' Lives' (1); this report introduces a 'top 10' key recommendations and encourages their implementation with audit (1); and it contains a chapter on 'near misses' (severe obstetric morbidity and complications) (1).

[It also contains a summary report of the United Kingdom Obstetric Surveillance System (UKOSS) for rare obstetric disorders.]

B

Four objectives of the report include: assessing the main causes of maternal deaths and identifying avoidable factors and substandard care (1); by doing the above, to improve care that pregnant and recently delivered women receive (1); to make recommendations to improve service provision (1); and to suggest areas for research and audit (1).

[Another objective is to produce a triennial report for England, Scotland, Wales and Northern Ireland.]

C

Direct maternal deaths are those caused by pregnancy or birth, e.g. haemorrhage or eclampsia (1). Indirect maternal deaths are those arising from a pre-existing or new medical or mental health condition aggravated by pregnancy, e.g. heart disease (1). Coincidental deaths are those that occur during pregnancy or within six weeks of birth unrelated to the patient being pregnant, e.g. road traffic accident or death from cancer (1). Late maternal deaths are those occurring between six weeks and one year after delivery (1). [The majority of late deaths are unrelated to pregnancy.]

D

The commonest cause of direct maternal death was thromboembolism and of indirect death cardiac disease (2). [Cardiac disease was the commonest cause of death overall.]

E ✓

The factors which appear to have contributed to the lack of decline in maternal mortality include: an increase in maternal age at childbirth (1), the rising number of women having babies who have been born outside the UK (migrants) (1); an increase in multiple births (which are associated with higher maternal mortality) (1); and health and lifestyle factors, e.g. obesity [more than half the mothers who died were overweight in the most recent report] and possibly female genital mutilation (1). Furthermore, there has been a steady increase in deaths of young mothers from diseases such as lung cancer and myocardial infarction, suggesting unhealthy lifestyle choices (1). A lack of basic clinical knowledge and skills, including resuscitation, among medical staff and a failure to identify common medical conditions or potential emergencies outside their immediate area of expertise has also contributed to this lack of reduction in maternal mortality (1).

[In conclusion, there has been an increase in the number of women whose social circumstances and health put them at an increased risk of maternal death.]

Further reading

Lewis G, ed. The Confidential Enquiry into Maternal and Child Health (CEMACH). *Saving Mothers' Lives: Reviewing Maternal Deaths to Make Motherhood Safer – 2003–2005*. The Seventh Report on Confidential Enquiries into Maternal Deaths in the United Kingdom. London: CEMACH, 2007.

1.1.27 Twin pregnancy

The incidence of twin pregnancy has gradually increased over the last decade.

A What complications are associated with twin pregnancies? (10 marks)
B What are the difficulties with antenatal screening for trisomy 21 in twin pregnancies? (5 marks)
C What complications are associated with the intrauterine death of one twin? (5 marks)

Key words in the question

- Incidence, twin pregnancy, increased.
- Complications.
- Difficulties, antenatal screening, trisomy 21, twin pregnancies.
- Complications, intrauterine death, one twin.

Essay plan

A

- Complications common to all pregnancies but higher in twins.
- Complications unique to twins/higher-order births.
- Maternal and fetal complications.

B
- Serum screening – the difficulties.
- NT – mono- and dichorionic.

C
- 'Vanishing twin syndrome' – no long-term effect on other twin.
- Late 2nd or 3rd trimester – cerebral palsy and increased neurological damage, death, preterm delivery.
- Coagulation disorder in the mother.

Suggested answer

A

Twin pregnancies are associated with an increase in the rate of miscarriage. Between 11 and 23 weeks, studies suggest 1%, 2% and 10% risk of miscarriage for singleton, dichorionic and monochorionic twin pregnancies (1). Some congenital anomalies are commoner in twins, including hydrocephalus, congenital heart disease and neural tube defects (1). Chromosomal defects are also more common, as many mothers of twins are in the older age group (1).

Preterm delivery is more common with twins (both iatrogenic and spontaneous) and about 30% of twin pregnancies deliver before 37 weeks. Prematurity is the major cause of perinatal morbidity and mortality (1). Maternal complications, including hyperemesis, anaemia, pre-eclampsia and gestational diabetes, are also more common (1). Twins also are associated with a higher incidence of placental abruption, placenta praevia, fetal malpresentation, stillbirths and neonatal death (1). [Identifying one or two of the maternal or fetal complications would be sufficient to gain the mark. The rest are included for completeness.]

Complications unique to twins or higher-order births include the in utero death of one twin (1), discordant growth of a twin (1), congenital anomalies specific to twin pregnancies, such as conjoined twins or twin reversed arterial perfusion (acardiac twin), and abnormalities related to the in utero environment, e.g. talipes and congenital dislocation of the hip (1).

A particular problem of monochorionic pregnancies is twin-to-twin transfusion syndrome, which is caused by arteriovenous communications between the two placentae (1). [Monochorionic twins have a higher complication rate than dichorionic twin pregnancies and are known to have four times higher perinatal mortality rates.]

B

Many mothers with a twin pregnancy are older (over 35 years) [due to an increase in dichorionic twins with maternal age and the impact of assisted conception]. Therefore screening for trisomy 21 is a common event but complex (1). Serum screening for Down syndrome is possible, and detection rates are better than using maternal age alone to decide who should be offered prenatal diagnostic tests. The level of serum markers is double the level expected in a singleton pregnancy. The test is further complicated in dichorionic twins where one is chromosomally normal. The normal twin's biochemistry masks the abnormal result in the affected twin, reducing the sensitivity of the test (2).

It is more usual to offer nuchal translucency (NT) screening (between 10 and 14 weeks) rather than serum screening in twin pregnancies (1). In dichorionic pregnancies, a risk of trisomy 21 is given for each fetus. In monochorionic twin pregnancies only one value is given (the mean of the two). This is the risk that both will have Down syndrome (1).

C

Up to 25% of pregnancies that are diagnosed as twin pregnancies in the first trimester continue as singleton pregnancies ('vanishing twin syndrome'). Very early loss of a twin does not seem to have a significant effect on the remaining twin (1).

Death of a twin late in the second trimester or in the third is a tragedy for the parents and poses a dilemma for the obstetrician (1). The surviving twin in both monochorionic and dichorionic pregnancies is at increased risk of neurological damage, cerebral palsy and death, although the risk in mono-chorionic pregnancy is three times higher (1). Most women will deliver within three weeks of the demise of the first twin, often resulting in prematurity, compounding the problems of the surviving twin (1). There is a potential risk of maternal coagulopathy in cases of prolonged retention of a dead fetus and a weekly coagulation screen is advisable (1).

[Loss of a twin late in the second trimester or in the third occurs in about 1% of cases. This may be due to severe growth restriction, fetal abnormalities or twin-to-twin transfusion syndrome.]

Further reading

Cameron A, Macara L, Brennand J, Milton P. *Fetal Medicine for the MRCOG and Beyond*. London: RCOG Press, 2002: 123–37.
Siddiqui F, McEwan A. Twins. *Obstetrics, Gynaecology and Reproductive Medicine* 2007; **17**: 289–95.

Gynaecology: Questions

1.2.1 Premenstrual syndrome

A 30-year-old patient presents with symptoms suggestive of premenstrual syndrome (PMS).

A Define PMS. (2 marks)

B How is PMS diagnosed? (2 marks)

C Outline the possible treatment regimes for the management of severe PMS. (10 marks)

D What is the role of gonadotrophin-releasing hormone analogues in treating PMS? (3 marks)

E When might surgery be appropriate for a woman with PMS? (3 marks)

1.2.2 Radiotherapy and chemotherapy

A Discuss the complications of radiotherapy. (10 marks)

B Discuss the complications which may occur in a patient undergoing chemotherapy for ovarian cancer. (10 marks)

1.2.3 Combined oral contraceptive pill

A A woman on a monophasic combined oral contraceptive pill (COCP) forgets to take it for two consecutive days. Counsel her appropriately. (6 marks)

B Mention five non-contraceptive benefits of the COCP. (5 marks)

C Discuss two drug interactions that can affect the efficacy of the COCP and give examples. (4 marks)

D How do progestogen-only contraceptive pills (POPs) exert their effect? Mention two advantages and two disadvantages. (5 marks)

1.2.4 Recurrent consecutive miscarriages

A 30-year-old woman attends the early-pregnancy assessment unit (EPAU) and is diagnosed with a silent (missed) first-trimester miscarriage. She is very upset, as she has had two other miscarriages, at 8 and 10 weeks, during the last year.

A Discuss the management of this woman's miscarriage. (7 marks)

B What investigations should be performed for recurrent miscarriages? (7 marks)

C How should a woman with antiphospholipid syndrome (APLS) be managed in her next pregnancy? (6 marks)

1.2.5 Dilemmas in contraception advice

A A 24-year-old on the combined oral contraceptive pill (COCP) attends your gynaecological clinic with migraines, which occur only towards the end of each packet of pills. She is normotensive, a non-smoker and has a normal body mass index (BMI). She wishes to continue with the COCP if possible because it has improved her heavy, painful periods. She requires effective contraception. How would you counsel this patient? (8 marks)

B A 37-year-old business executive, who smokes 15 cigarettes a day, attends the gynaecology outpatient department for contraceptive advice. She uses condoms for contraception and wishes to switch to a more convenient and effective method. She wants to retain her fertility but does not wish to become pregnant at present. Counsel her regarding her options. (12 marks)

1.2.6 Cornual pregnancy

A 25-year-old woman attends the emergency gynaecology unit at 11 weeks' gestation. She complains of right-sided pelvic pain. A departmental ultrasound scan is suggestive of a cornual pregnancy.

A What is a cornual pregnancy and how is it diagnosed? (5 marks)

B The patient wants expectant management, as she wishes to avoid surgery. How might she be persuaded against this modality of treatment? (5 marks)

C What are the contraindications to medical treatment? (5 marks)

D What advice should she be given for management of any future pregnancies? (5 marks)

1.2.7 Menorrhagia – fibroid uterus

A 41-year-old woman with very heavy regular periods attends the gynaecological outpatient department. The fundus of her uterus is palpable abdominally, approximating to 16 weeks' gestational size.

A What investigations would you perform and why? (4 marks)

B You discover she has a large single fibroid 12 cm in diameter. Discuss non-medical treatment options, including complications. (15 marks)

C Having considered the options, she desires medical treatment. What are her options? (1 mark)

1.2.8 Dysmenorrhoea

A Define dysmenorrhoea and distinguish between primary and secondary dysmenorrhoea. (3 marks)

B Outline the typical clinical features of primary and secondary dysmenorrhoea. (8 marks)

C What are appropriate treatment options for primary dysmenorrhoea? (7 marks)

D Briefly outline the role of prostaglandins in primary dysmenorrhoea. (2 marks)

1.2.9 Silent (missed) miscarriage

A primigravid woman attends the booking clinic at 11 weeks' gestation. An ultrasound examination reveals a silent (missed) miscarriage.

A What are the different management options for this woman? Give two advantages and two disadvantages for each method. (9 marks)

B The woman chooses to have surgery. Discuss this procedure. (7 marks)

C Outline optimal postoperative management. (4 marks)

1.2.10 Cancer of the fallopian tube

Consider a woman presenting with cancer of the fallopian tube.

A Discuss the predisposing and protective factors. (4 marks)

B What types of cancer are found in primary disease? (4 marks)

C What are the presenting symptoms, including the classical presentation, and how is the diagnosis generally made? (4 marks)

D Outline the FIGO staging of fallopian tube carcinoma. (8 marks)

1.2.11 Endometrial cancer

Mrs Smith is a 64-year-old woman who presents with a solitary episode of postmenopausal bleeding lasting four days.

A What investigations would you perform to confirm or exclude endometrial cancer? (5 marks)

B Assuming a diagnosis of endometrial cancer, how can you assess the disease extent before surgery? (5 marks)

C How is endometrial cancer staged? Describe stage III disease. (6 marks)

D What are the common indications for post-hysterectomy radiotherapy? (4 marks)

1.2.12 Hormone replacement therapy

A 49-year-old woman with an intact uterus presents with hot flushes, night sweats and 12 months of amenorrhoea. She requests hormone replacement therapy (HRT).

A How should she be counselled? (10 marks)

B What types of HRT may be suitable for her and why? (5 marks)

C Summarize the non-oestrogen-based treatments available. (5 marks)

1.2.13 Subfertility

A 32-year-old woman attends the fertility clinic with her partner. They have a two-year history of subfertility.

A What aspects of the history and examination should be ascertained at this consultation? (13 marks)

B What investigations may be useful in order to establish the cause of their subfertility? (4 marks)

C What lifestyle advice should be given to this couple to enhance their chances of conception? (3 marks)

1.2.14 Vulval cancer

A Discuss the incidence, age group affected and predisposing factors associated with vulval cancer. What is the commonest type of tumour? (5 marks)

B Outline the FIGO staging of this disease. (7 marks)

C How would you treat a stage Ia tumour? (2 marks)

D What are the complications associated with vulval and inguinal surgery? (6 marks)

1.2.15 Laparoscopy

You have decided to perform diagnostic laparoscopy for pelvic pain.

A What are the relevant points that should be discussed at the time of taking consent? (Do not include anaesthetic complications.) (11 marks)

B Discuss a safe closed-entry laparoscopic technique. (9 marks)

1.2.16 Overactive bladder syndrome

A 62-year-old woman attends your gynaecology clinic with symptoms of overactive bladder syndrome (OABS).

A Outline the characteristics associated with OABS. (4 marks)

B Discuss the treatments that may be offered to this patient, assuming the diagnosis of OABS. (10 marks)

C What are the main complications associated with the surgical treatment of OABS? (6 marks)

1.2.17 Polycystic ovarian syndrome

A 31-year-old woman attends the gynaecological outpatient clinic with a three-year history of oligomenorrhoea and hirsutism. Her body mass index (BMI) is 38 kg/m². You suspect she has polycystic ovarian syndrome (PCOS).

A How would you confirm the diagnosis of PCOS? (5 marks)

B Assuming the diagnosis is PCOS, how would you counsel this patient? (15 marks)

1.2.18 Complications of postvaginal hysterectomy

You are the registrar on call and you are asked to see a 66-year-old, well-controlled hypertensive woman who has had a vaginal hysterectomy with pelvic floor repair four hours ago. She has a blood pressure of 70/50 mmHg and pulse of 138 beats per minute.

A What features would you look for on clinical examination? (6 marks)

B What is the likely diagnosis? (1 mark)

C Justify your investigations. (3 marks)

D Outline your further management. (10 marks)

1.2.19 Acute pelvic inflammatory disease

A 19-year-old girl is referred with a three-day history of lower abdominal pain and tenderness and offensive vaginal discharge. She has been sexually active with her current partner for one month.

A What other features would suggest a diagnosis of acute pelvic inflammatory disease (PID)? (3 marks)

B If the diagnosis was uncertain, what three investigations would be the most helpful? (3 marks)

C Assuming moderate PID is confirmed, outline a suitable management plan. (7 marks)

D When should patients with acute PID be admitted to hospital? (3 marks)

E When should surgical treatment be considered? Mention three possible methods. (4 marks)

1.2.20 Postmenopausal ovarian cyst

A 63-year-old postmenopausal woman is referred to the gynaecological clinic by her general practitioner with an ovarian cyst 5 cm in diameter apparent on transabdominal ultrasound scan.

A What investigations are appropriate in this case and why? (6 marks)

B If results of these investigations suggest that the patient has a very low risk (<3%) of having ovarian cancer, outline your management. (9 marks)

C If investigations reveal a high risk of ovarian cancer, how should she be managed? (5 marks)

1.2.21 Emergency contraception and laparoscopic clip sterilization

A Identify two methods of emergency contraception. When would you prescribe it and what advice would you give to a patient receiving emergency contraception? (13 marks)

B What factors are important in counselling a woman in the outpatient clinic requesting laparoscopic clip sterilization? Do not discuss specific risks associated with laparoscopy. (7 marks)

1.2.22 Stress urinary incontinence

A 45-year-old woman with a body mass index (BMI) of 35 kg/m^2 presents to the gynaecology clinic with symptoms suggestive of stress urinary incontinence (SUI). She has had no treatment from her general practitioner.

A What information would help you to make a diagnosis of 'pure' stress incontinence? (12 marks)

B Assuming a diagnosis of 'pure' stress incontinence in this case, what would be your immediate management plan (non-surgical)? Explain why and how and over what timescale it would be given. (8 marks)

1.2.23 Cervical cancer

A patient is referred to the gynaecology clinic with possible cervical cancer.

A Where should this patient be seen? What findings would raise the index of suspicion of cervical cancer? How would you confirm the diagnosis? (5 marks)

B The diagnosis is confirmed as stage Ib cervical cancer. What is stage Ib cervical cancer? Discuss the options for treatment in this situation. (11 marks)

C What post-treatment support and follow-up are required? (4 marks)

1.2.24 Ovarian hyperstimulation syndrome

A 36-year-old woman undergoing in vitro fertilization (IVF) treatment is admitted with severe abdominal pain and vomiting.

A Excluding ovarian hyperstimulation syndrome (OHSS), what differential diagnoses should be considered in this woman? (3 marks)

B Discuss how OHSS is classified. (9 marks)

C In this case justify your examination and any investigations you may wish to perform. (8 marks)

1.2.25 Chronic pelvic pain

A Define chronic pelvic pain. (2 marks)

B How would you manage a patient with chronic pelvic pain? (18 marks)

Gynaecology: Answers

1.2.1   Premenstrual syndrome

A 30-year-old patient presents with symptoms suggestive of premenstrual syndrome (PMS).

A   Define PMS. (2 marks)

B   How is PMS diagnosed? (2 marks)

C   Outline the possible treatment regimes for the management of severe PMS. (10 marks)

D   What is the role of gonadotrophin-releasing hormone analogues in treating PMS? (3 marks)

E   When might surgery be appropriate for a woman with PMS? (3 marks)

Key words in the question

- 30-year-old, premenstrual syndrome.
- Define PMS.
- Treatment regimes.
- Role, gonadotrophin-releasing hormone analogues.
- Surgery.

Essay plan

A

- Physical, psychological and behavioural symptoms.

B

- Symptoms recorded prospectively over two cycles using a symptom diary.

C

- First, second, third and fourth line.

D

- Only for severe cases.
- Six months only − longer with add-back.

E

- TAH + BSO − first trial of GnRHa with HRT including testosterone.

Suggested answer

A

Premenstrual syndrome (PMS) is the occurrence of distressing physical, behavioural and psychological symptoms in the absence of organic or psychiatric disease; the symptoms recur during the luteal phase of the menstrual cycle and regresses by the end of menstruation (2).

B

The diagnosis is made following prospective recording over two cycles using a symptom diary. Typical psychological symptoms include mood swings, irritability, depression; physical symptoms include breast tenderness and bloating; behavioural symptoms include reduced cognitive ability and an increase in accidents (2).

C

An integrated approach is beneficial. This may include complementary therapies, such as evening primrose oil, which often have no evidence base (1). First-line therapy includes advising exercise, cognitive-behavioural therapy, combined new-generation pills such as Yasmin or continuous or luteal-phase low-dose selective serotonin reuptake inhibitors (SSRIs) (2). Second-line treatment includes oestradiol patches with the levonorgestrel-containing intrauterine system (Mirena) or luteal-phase oral progestogens (3). If this fails, then third-line treatment with gonadotrophin-releasing hormone analogue (GnRHa) with add-back hormone replacement therapy (HRT), e.g. tibolone, will suppress ovarian function and abolish PMS symptoms (2). Occasionally hysterectomy and bilateral salpingo-oophorectomy (BSO) is undertaken, and oestrogen and sometimes testosterone replacement may be required (2).

D

Due to its hypo-oestrogenic effect GnRHa should be used only in cases of severe PMS. Although not licensed for treating PMS, it is a very effective treatment (1). Add-back therapy such as tibolone or continuous combined HRT is recommended, as it reduces menopausal symptoms without the reappearance of PMS-like progestogenic effects. Furthermore, bone mineral density can be maintained by using HRT. Treatment with a GnRHa is normally continued for six months only. Patients on long-term treatment (more than six months) should take HRT and have annual measurements of bone mineral density (2).

E

In severe PMS hysterectomy and BSO is beneficial, as it permanently suppresses ovulation (1). Most patients do not require surgery as a satisfactory alternative can usually be found. Any woman contemplating total abdominal hysterectomy and BSO should have a trial of GnRHa (to ensure symptoms disappear) and have HRT to ensure it is tolerated. If the woman is less than 50 years old (as is the case with this patient) oestrogen and testosterone replacement should be considered (2).

Further reading

Royal College of Obstetricians and Gynaecologists. *Management of Premenstrual Syndrome.* Green-Top Guideline No. 48. London: RCOG, December 2007.

1.2.2 Radiotherapy and chemotherapy

A Discuss the complications of radiotherapy. (10 marks)

B Discuss the complications which may occur in a patient undergoing chemotherapy for ovarian cancer. (10 marks)

Key words in the question

- Discuss, complications, radiotherapy.
- Discuss, complications, chemotherapy, ovarian cancer.

Essay plan

A

- Acute and late, skin, urinary tract, bowel, ovaries, vagina.

B

- Blood, bowel, genitourinary, neuro, liver.

Suggested answer

A

The complications of radiotherapy can be subdivided into acute and late.

Acute toxicity occurs as a result of loss of surface epithelial cells, and consequently recovery occurs in a matter of days or weeks following the cessation of treatment (1). In the skin this may cause localized erythema and desquamation (1). In the bowel this may give rise to diarrhoea (1). In the bladder urinary frequency and dysuria can occur (1). Effects on bone marrow may result in anaemia, neutropenia and thrombocytopenia (1).

Late radiotherapy damage can occur months or even years after treatment. Bowel effects include acute or subacute obstruction, bleeding, perforation, fistula formation and malabsorption (1). The bladder may be affected long term due to contracture formation, with associated reduction in bladder capacity. Haemorrhagic cystitis may occur, causing haematuria and pain. Fistula formation can occur, especially with the vagina and ureteric obstruction, and hydronephrosis has been described (2). In premenopausal women pelvic irradiation can cause subsequent ovarian failure and premature menopause (1). Vaginal effects include atrophy, causing shortening and stenosis. Vaginal dryness can occur, which may lead to sexual problems (1).

B

Complications of chemotherapy are best discussed by the system affected. Haematologically, myelosuppression is common with platinum-based chemotherapy such as carboplatin. This causes anaemia, thrombocytopenia and granulocytopenia, resulting in an increased risk of spontaneous bleeding and infection (2). Gastrointestinal effects include nausea, vomiting and ulceration of the intestinal tract. This can cause pain and dysphagia when the mouth and oesophagus are affected and diarrhoea and necrotizing enterocolitis when the large intestine is affected (2). Cisplatin can cause renal tubular toxicity and therefore acute renal failure. Haemorrhagic cystitis may occur due to the irritative effect of some chemotherapeutic metabolites, particularly those of cyclophosphamide (2). Neurotoxicity can occur with different chemotherapeutic agents. Cisplatin causes ototoxicity, peripheral neuropathy and, rarely, blindness (2). Paclitaxel can also cause peripheral sensory neuropathy, which may worsen when it is used in combination with cisplatin (1). Hepatotoxicity can occur, with associated elevation of liver enzymes (1).

Further reading

Luesley D, Achesen N, eds. *Gynaecological Oncology for the MRCOG and Beyond*. London: RCOG Press, 2004.

1.2.3 Combined oral contraceptive pill

A A woman on a monophasic combined oral contraceptive pill (COCP) forgets to take it for two consecutive days. Counsel her appropriately. (6 marks)

B Mention five non-contraceptive benefits of the COCP. (5 marks)

C Discuss two drug interactions that can affect the efficacy of the COCP and give examples. (4 marks)

D How do progestogen-only contraceptive pills (POPs) exert their effect? Mention two advantages and two disadvantages. (5 marks)

Key words in the question

- Monophasic, COCP, forgets, two days, counsel.
- Five non-contraceptive benefits.
- Two drug interactions, examples.
- POPs, effect, two advantages, two disadvantages.

Essay plan

A

- Establish if 20 μg or 30/35 μg pill.
- 30/35 μg – no problem.
- 20 μg – condoms for next seven days. Additional risk pregnancy depending on where she is in her cycle.

B

- Reduced menstrual loss, PID, ovarian/endometrial cancer, dysmenorrhoea, ectopic pregnancy reduced.

C

- Enzyme inducers, e.g. anticonvulsants and rifampicin.
- Enterohepatic circulation, e.g. some broad-spectrum antibiotics.

D

- POP – effects on cervical mucus, endometrium and ovulation.
- Advantages – breast-feeding and useful when oestrogen contraindicated.
- Disadvantages – irregular bleeding and must take it at same time every day.

Suggested answer

A

I would ascertain whether she is on a 20 μg or a 30/35 μg ethinyl oestradiol pill (1). If she is taking a higher-dose pill (30 μg or 35 μg), she should take a pill as soon as possible and continue taking one pill daily as normal. She does not require any further contraceptive protection (1).

If she is on a lower-dose pill (20 μg), she should take her next pill as soon as possible and continue taking further pills daily as normal (1). However, she needs additional contraceptive protection, e.g. condoms, or she could avoid sexual intercourse until she has taken pills for seven consecutive days (1). If she missed the pills in the first week of her cycle (after the pill-free week) and had unprotected intercourse, she would reduce her risk of pregnancy by using emergency contraception (1). If she missed the pills during the third week, she should finish the packet and commence the next packet of pills the following day. By doing so she will not require emergency contraception but will not have a withdrawal bleed that cycle (1).

B

Five non-contraceptive benefits of the COCP are reduced menstrual blood loss (1), a reduction in pelvic inflammatory disease (1), a lower risk of ovarian and endometrial cancer (1), a reduction in risk of ectopic pregnancy (1) and less dysmenorrhoea (1). [Other non-contraceptive benefits include a reduction in benign breast disease, less chance of functional ovarian cysts and fewer premenstrual syndrome symptoms.]

C

Two drug interactions that reduce the efficacy of COCP are drugs that induce liver enzymes (1) and medications that affect the enterohepatic circulation (1). Many anticonvulsants, e.g. carbamazepine, phenytoin, and antitubercle antibiotics, e.g. rifampicin and rifabutin, accelerate the metabolism and elimination of oestrogen and progestogen. For a short course of an enzyme-inducing drug, the dose of oestrogen in the COCP should be increased to 50 μg daily (unlicensed). For longer courses of enzyme-inducing drugs, an alternative method should be used, e.g. copper intrauterine device (1).

Some antibiotics, e.g. ampicillin and doxycycline, impair the bacterial flora responsible for recycling ethinyl oestradiol from the large bowel. Additional precautions, e.g. condoms, should be taken while the woman is on the antibiotic and for seven days after stopping it (1). [If the antibiotic course exceeds three weeks, the additional precautions are no longer required because the flora develops antibacterial resistance.]

D

Progestogen-only contraceptive pills (POPs) are believed to exert their effect by a combination of rendering cervical mucus hostile to sperm, a reduction in ovulation (Cerazette inhibits ovulation in over 95% of cycles) and a reduction in the receptivity of endometrium to implantation (1).

Two advantages of the POP are that it is a useful contraceptive for breast-feeding mothers (1) [it has no effect on quality or quantity of milk production] and it can be safely used in patients for whom oestrogen is contraindicated (1) [history of venous thromboembolism, smoker >35 years old, hypertension >140/90 mmHg, migraine with aura, etc. POPs have a lower dose of progestogen than COCPs so they have fewer progestogenic side effects].

Two disadvantages include irregular bleeding (1) and the need to take the POP at the same time every day (1). [If she is more than three hours late in taking the POP, then she should use condoms for the next two days as well as taking the POP at the correct time. Cerazette is similar to COCPs in that the rules for missed pills commence after 12 hours.]

Further reading

Combined hormonal contraceptives, sections 7.3.1 and 7.3.2. *British National Formulary* (BNF), No. 52, March 2008: 415–22.
Webberley H, Mann M. Oral contraception – updated. *Current Obstetrics and Gynaecology* 2006; **16**: 21–9.

1.2.4 Recurrent consecutive miscarriages

A 30-year-old woman attends the early-pregnancy assessment unit (EPAU) and is diagnosed with a silent (missed) first-trimester miscarriage. She is very upset, as she has had two other miscarriages, at 8 and 10 weeks, during the last year.

A Discuss the management of this woman's miscarriage. (7 marks)

B What investigations should be performed for recurrent miscarriages? (7 marks)

C How should a woman with antiphospholipid syndrome (APLS) be managed in her next pregnancy? (6 marks)

Key words in the question

- Silent, miscarriage.
- Two other miscarriages.
- Discuss, management, miscarriage.
- Investigations, recurrent miscarriages.
- How, APLS, managed, next pregnancy.

Essay plan

A

- Empathy with patient.
- Management options – expectant, medical, surgical.
- Karyotyping of POC.

B

- Karyotyping of couple.
- Check for thrombophilias.
- Ascertain normal uterine anatomy.

C

- Psychological support.
- Combination of aspirin and heparin treatment.
- Psychological support and USS.
- Close monitoring of pregnancy because of increased risks of complications – pre-eclampsia, IUGR.

Suggested answer

A

This woman is understandably upset and should be treated with empathy and sympathy (1). Management options for a silent miscarriage should be discussed with her. Expectant management avoids intervention but may take a few weeks for the products to be expelled (1). Medical management with oral and vaginal prostaglandins is very effective in about 80% of cases and means that surgery may be avoided (1). The patient should be advised to return to hospital if heavy bleeding or pain occurs (1). The alternative would be to have surgical evacuation of retained products of conception after cervical ripening (1). This would complete the procedure on the same day but would involve hospital admission and anaesthetic (1). The products of conception should be sent for karyotyping, as this helps with counselling for future pregnancies (1).

B

As this patient has had three recurrent consecutive miscarriages, she warrants investigation (1). Parental karyotyping should be performed, as 3–5% of recurrent miscarriage patients will have a balanced structural chromosomal anomaly such as Robertsonian translocation (1). Investigation for inherited thrombophilias such as protein C or S deficiency should be arranged (1). Antiphospholipid syndrome (APLS) is found in 15% of recurrent miscarriages (1). Moderate to high titres of lupus anticoagulant or anticardiolipin antibody need to be obtained six weeks apart to confirm this diagnosis (1). An ultrasound scan to check for uterine anomalies must be performed (1). If any subsequent pregnancy fails, cytogenic analysis of the products of conception should be performed (1).

C

An untreated woman with APLS has only a 10% chance of spontaneously delivering a baby at term due to thrombotic episodes, especially in the placenta. She should therefore be treated with thromboprophylaxis (1). The patient is advised to take low-dose aspirin as soon as a positive pregnancy test is obtained. This alone increases the success of the pregnancy to 40% (1). When taken along with low-molecular-weight heparin once a day, the success of achieving a full-term pregnancy is increased to 70% (1). As this is a high-risk pregnancy, the woman's antenatal care should be led by a consultant (1). In the earlier part of the pregnancy she needs regular visits to the early-pregnancy assessment unit (EPAU) for psychological support and ultrasound scans (1). Regular antenatal visits are needed, as these pregnancies are at a higher risk of pre-eclampsia, intrauterine growth restriction and preterm birth (1).

Further reading

Royal College of Obstetricians and Gynaecologists. *The Investigation and Treatment of Couples with Recurrent Miscarriages.* Green-Top Guideline No. 17. London: RCOG, May 2003.

1.2.5 Dilemmas in contraception advice

A A 24-year-old on the combined oral contraceptive pill (COCP) attends your gynaecological clinic with migraines, which occur only towards the end of each packet of pills. She is normotensive, a non-smoker and has a normal body mass index (BMI). She wishes to continue with the COCP if possible because it has improved her heavy, painful periods. She requires effective contraception. How would you counsel this patient? (8 marks)

B A 37-year-old business executive, who smokes 15 cigarettes a day, attends the gynaecology outpatient department for contraceptive advice. She uses condoms for contraception and wishes to switch to a more convenient and effective method. She wants to retain her fertility but does not wish to become pregnant at present. Counsel her regarding her options. (12 marks)

Key words in the question

A
- 24-year-old, COCP, migraines, normotensive, non-smoker, normal BMI.
- Heavy painful periods, effective contraception, counsel.

B
- 37-year-old, smokes, contraceptive advice.
- Effective method.
- Retain, fertility, counsel.

Essay plan

A
- Identify pill type.
- Type of migraine.
- Focal aura – stop pill.
- Alternative methods – Mirena, Depo-Provera.

B
- COCP contraindicated.
- All POPs suitable.
- Best option probably LARCs except Depo-Provera.
- Verbal, written information, follow-up appointment if needs more time to decide.

Suggested answer

A

I would ascertain which pill the patient is taking. Triphasic pills contain variable oestrogen doses and may cause premenstrual-like symptoms during the last week of the packet. Symptoms include headache, irritability and bloating (1).

The type of migraines the woman experiences are important (1). Migraine with aura (focal neurological symptoms) is associated with a much higher increased risk [approximately fivefold] of ischaemic stroke and is an absolute contraindication to taking the combined oral contraceptive pill (COCP) (1). [Neurological symptoms can be visual or sensory. Visual symptoms are the commonest – a visual aura is typically a bright spot, which increases in size to form the letter 'C' with zigzags. It often lasts for up to an hour and precedes the headache. Generalized 'flashing lights', blurred vision and photophobia are common in migraine sufferers and do not suggest focal ischaemia.]

If this patient's migraines are not associated with focal aura, I would advise her to take a monophasic pill continuously for three months before having a withdrawal bleed (tricycling) (1).

If this woman has focal aura, I would strongly advise her to discontinue the COCP (1). If she has migraine without focal symptoms and does not require ergot derivatives for treatment, she can continue the COCP with caution (1). She should have regular assessments for arterial risk factors, e.g. hypertension and smoking. If the migraines increase in severity or frequency, it is sensible to stop the COCP (1).

Alternative suitable contraceptive methods include Mirena or Depo-Provera. Both methods may result in very light periods or amenorrhoea, thereby improving or even abolishing this woman's menorrhagia and dysmenorrhoea (1). [All progestogen-only methods could be used, as none carry an increased risk of ischaemic stroke, although Mirena and Depo-Provera offer the best chance of reducing her menorrhagia and dysmenorrhoea.]

B

Since this woman is older than 35 years and smokes cigarettes, the combined oral contraceptive pill (COCP) is contraindicated (1). All progestogen-only pills (POPs) can be considered, although as a busy business executive she may find it hard to remember to take the pills within the three-hour window (1). Cerazette® is a very effective POP with a 12-hour 'missed pill' rule and so may appeal to this woman (1). Perhaps the best option is long-acting reversible contraception (LARC) such as Mirena, copper intrauterine device (CuIUD) or Implanon (3). Since she wishes to retain her fertility and is 37 years old, I would not suggest Depo-Provera®, as it is associated with a delayed return of fertility of up to a year (1).

I would give verbal and written information on the benefits, failure rates, side effects and risks and when to seek advice regarding LARC methods (3). Mirena, Implanon and CuIUDs are rapidly reversible, so would all be suitable for this patient (1). [Mirena is licensed for five years, Implanon for three years and CuIUDs between 5 and 10 years.] Should the patient feel she needs more time to decide which method she wishes to use, I would arrange a follow-up appointment for her, and exclude pregnancy before inserting/fitting the LARC (1).

Further reading

National Institute for Health and Clinical Excellence. *Long-Acting Reversible Contraception*. NICE Clinical Guideline No. 30. London: NICE, October 2005.

Progestogen-only contraceptives, and Contraceptive devices, sections 7.3.2 and 7.3.4. *British National Formulary* (BNF), No. 52, March 2008: 421–4.

Szarewski A. Choice of contraception. *Current Obstetrics and Gynaecology* 2006; **16**: 361–5.

1.2.6 Cornual pregnancy

A 25-year-old woman attends the emergency gynaecology unit at 11 weeks' gestation. She complains of right-sided pelvic pain. A departmental ultrasound scan is suggestive of a cornual pregnancy.

A What is a cornual pregnancy and how is it diagnosed? (5 marks)

B The patient wants expectant management as she wishes to avoid surgery. How might she be persuaded against this modality of treatment? (5 marks)

C What are the contraindications to medical treatment? (5 marks)

D What advice should she be given for management of any future pregnancies? (5 marks)

Key words in the question

- 11 weeks' gestation, cornual pregnancy.
- What, cornual pregnancy.
- How, diagnosed.
- Wants expectant management.
- How, persuaded against, treatment.
- What, contraindications to medical treatment.
- Advice, future pregnancies.

Essay plan

A

- Definition.
- Ultrasound criteria.
- Laparoscopic diagnosis.

B

- Expectant not recommended.
- Explain life-threatening risks.
- Discuss medical treatment.

C

- Absolute contraindications – unstable patient, ruptured ectopic, allergy to methotrexate.
- Relative contraindications – large ectopic, heartbeat.
- Needs follow-up.

D

- Early assessment of pregnancy site.
- Mode of delivery – caesarean section.

Suggested answer

A

A pregnancy located in the interstitial part of the fallopian tube is defined as a cornual pregnancy (1). Transvaginal ultrasound scan (TVS) is the main modality used for diagnosis. The criterion used is an empty uterus with a gestational sac seen separately and less than 1 cm from the most lateral edge of the uterine cavity. The sac is surrounded by a thin myometrial layer and can be confused with an eccentrically placed intrauterine gestational sac, making the diagnosis difficult (2). When there is a strong suspicion of extrauterine pregnancy and the diagnosis is not confirmed by ultrasound, laparoscopy should be performed (1). The distension of the cornua of the uterus distorting the normal shape will then be suggestive of a cornual pregnancy (1).

B

The patient should be informed that expectant management is not a recommended modality of treatment for cornual pregnancy, as there is a high chance of sudden uterine rupture with significant intraperitoneal bleeding (1). This may lead to hysterectomy (1). The condition may be life-threatening if surgery is not immediately available. Mortality rates of 2.0–2.5% have been reported (1). The patient's concerns regarding treatment must be explored to identify why she is reluctant to have treatment. Medical treatment with systemic methotrexate is safe and highly effective (1). Surgical intervention can be avoided in the majority of women. The patient has to be convinced of the need of regular outpatient monitoring and that she must return to hospital in case of pain or bleeding (1).

C

Medical treatment should not be initiated in a haemodynamically unstable patient or where there is evidence of rupture of the cornua (1). The patient should not have any medical contraindication to the use of methotrexate (1). A large ectopic pregnancy and the presence of a heartbeat are also relative contraindications (2). Regular follow-up is essential and therefore if the patient is not motivated or does not have the facility for attending hospital in an emergency, inpatient treatment may be required (1).

D

Since there is a recognized recurrence risk of ectopic pregnancy, including cornual pregnancy, the patient should be advised to attend the early pregnancy assessment unit as soon as she discovers she is pregnant (1). This is to allow the location of the pregnancy via TVS (1). Although cornual pregnancy is difficult to diagnose at an early gestation, follow-up may allow earlier intervention (1). There is no definitive guidance of the optimum mode of delivery in a future pregnancy. However, the risk of uterine rupture is well documented (1). The consensus of opinion is to deliver by caesarean section after surgical or medical management of a cornual pregnancy (1).

Further reading

Faraj R, Steel M. Management of cornual (interstitial) pregnancy. *The Obstetrician and Gynaecologist* 2007; **9**: 249–55.

1.2.7   Menorrhagia – fibroid uterus

A 41-year-old woman with very heavy regular periods attends the gynaecological outpatient department. The fundus of her uterus is palpable abdominally, approximating to 16 weeks' gestational size.

A   What investigations would you perform and why? (4 marks)

B   You discover she has a large single fibroid 12 cm in diameter. Discuss non-medical treatment options, including complications. (15 marks)

C   Having considered the options, she desires medical treatment. What are her options? (1 mark)

Key words in the question

- 41-year-old, heavy regular periods, uterus, palpable, 16 weeks' gestational size.
- Investigations, why.
- Large single fibroid, treatment options, complications.
- Desires medical treatment, options.

Essay plan

A

- FBC, U + Es, USS, CA125.

B

- Surgical – UAE, myomectomy, hysterectomy.
- Complications, side effects.

C

- Medical treatment.
- UAE, myomectomy, appropriate counselling.

Suggested answer

A

I would arrange a full blood count (FBC) to exclude iron deficiency anaemia (1) and urea and electrolytes (U + Es) to ensure normal renal function, as a large pelvic mass may occasionally cause ureteric obstruction, with hydronephrosis or even renal failure (1). An ultrasound scan would likely confirm whether the mass was a fibroid or ovarian cyst (1). In uncertain cases a magnetic resonance imaging (MRI) scan may be helpful, and if the mass is ovarian, the cancer antigen 125 (CA125) level should be measured, as it is elevated in 80% of epithelial ovarian cancers (1).

B

Non-medical options include uterine artery embolization (UAE). If there are symptoms of pain and pressure from the pelvic mass and the woman wishes to retain her uterus, UAE is a suitable option (1). The blood supply to the uterus is blocked and this causes the fibroids to shrink. Potentially, fertility is retained but this cannot be guaranteed (1). Common side effects include persistent vaginal discharge and post-embolization syndrome (pain, nausea, vomiting and fever) (1). Less common is premature ovarian failure and haematoma (1). Very rarely, septicaemia may occur, necessitating hysterectomy (1).

Surgical options include myomectomy. This involves the surgical removal (usually via laparotomy) of the large fibroid. Fibroids have a false capsule and can usually be enucleated ('shelled out') at surgery (1). Pre-treatment with gonadotrophin-releasing hormone analogue (GnRHa) to reduce the size of the fibroid and the blood loss at surgery is often given (1). Complications of myomectomy include adhesion development, pain, impaired fertility, recurrence of fibroids and hysterectomy if the bleeding during the procedure was uncontrollable (2).

The other surgical option is hysterectomy. This would cure the menorrhagia and remove the mass in the abdomen (1). Hysterectomy removes her fertility and the patient needs to accept this prior to surgery (1). The risks associated with hysterectomy include infection, intraoperative haemorrhage (increased risk with fibroids), risk of damage to urinary tract and bowel, and the rare risk of thrombosis (2). The pros and cons of removing the ovaries at the time of hysterectomy should be discussed and the woman supported in making an informed decision (1). The benefits and risks of HRT, should she opt for a bilateral salpingo-oophorectomy, need to be discussed (1).

C

The medical options include treatment with Mirena, tranexamic acid, non-steroidals, oral progestogens for three weeks in every month, and GnRHa. However, these are likely to provide only temporary relief at best (1).

Further reading

National Institute for Health and Clinical Excellence. *Heavy Menstrual Bleeding*. Clinical Guideline No. 44. London: NICE, January 2007.

1.2.8 Dysmenorrhoea

A Define dysmenorrhoea and distinguish between primary and secondary dysmenorrhoea. (3 marks)

B Outline the typical clinical features of primary and secondary dysmenorrhoea. (8 marks)

C What are appropriate treatment options for primary dysmenorrhoea? (7 marks)

D Briefly outline the role of prostaglandins in primary dysmenorrhoea. (2 marks)

Key words in the question

- Define, dysmenorrhoea, distinguish, primary, secondary.
- Outline, features, primary, secondary dysmenorrhoea.
- Appropriate treatment, primary.
- Outline, role, prostaglandins, primary.

Essay plan

A

- Definition, primary and secondary.

B

- Primary – adolescent, spasmodic pain, nausea and vomiting, no pathology.
- Secondary – 30–45, bloating, backache, pelvic pathology.

C

- Reassure, analgesia, NSAIDs, paracetamol, co-proxamol, COCP.

D

- Increased myometrial activity, excess production of PGs/PGF$_{2\alpha}$.

Suggested answer

A

Dysmenorrhoea is excessive menstrual pain that is severe enough to limit normal activities or require medication (1). Primary dysmenorrhoea is menstrual pain occurring in the absence of uterine or pelvic pathology (1). In secondary dysmenorrhoea there is an identifiable underlying pathology, e.g. endometriosis or pelvic inflammatory disease (1).

B

Primary dysmenorrhoea usually occurs in young women with ovulatory cycles shortly after the menarche (1). Typically the girl complains of spasmodic cramping pain, occurring just before or during menstruation, radiating to the back and down her thighs, which lasts for approximately 48 hours. Menstrual bleeding is often normal and pain can be severe even when the period is light (1). Associated symptoms include nausea and vomiting, lower backache, diarrhoea and headache (1). Pelvic examination is negative in cases of primary dysmenorrhoea, although if the patient is not sexually active a rectal examination or abdominal ultrasound scan may be preferred (1).

Patients with secondary dysmenorrhoea are frequently older, often between 30 and 45 years (1). Their pain is usually associated with abdominal bloating and backache and increases progressively in the luteal phase, being maximal at the onset of menstruation (1). Abdominopelvic examination findings will vary according to the cause but may include a tender and/or an enlarged uterus, tender or fixed adnexal masses and nodules of endometriosis palpable on the uterosacral ligaments and cervicitis with mucopurulent discharge (2). [Occasionally secondary dysmenorrhoea occurs in adolescents and is most often due to endometriosis.]

C

Patients with primary dysmenorrhoea usually respond to reassurance and non-steroidal anti-inflammatory drugs (NSAIDs) such as ibuprofen or naproxen (2). An equivalent to 600 mg of ibuprofen four times daily commencing one day prior to the onset of menstruation until day 2 or 3 is recommended (2). Paracetamol and co-proxamol are less effective than ibuprofen or naproxen but may be considered if NSAIDs are contraindicated (1). The combined oral contraceptive pill (COCP) is commonly used for primary dysmenorrhoea if NSAIDs are ineffective or contraindicated (1). More than 90% of adolescent girls have significant pain reduction within three months of commencing a COCP (1).

D

Primary dysmenorrhoea is associated with increased myometrial activity in the uterus induced by excess production of prostaglandins (1). There are increased circulating levels of prostaglandin (PG) F$_{2\alpha}$ in women with dysmenorrhoea. PGF$_{2\alpha}$ is a potent myometrial vasoconstrictor and intrauterine pressure is significantly higher in dysmenorrhoea (1).

Further reading

Raine-Fenning N. Dysmenorrhoea. *Current Obstetrics and Gynaecology* 2005; **15**: 394–401.
Siddiqui N, Pitkin J. Menstrual disturbances. *Obstetrics, Gynaecology and Reproductive Medicine* 2007; **17**: 154–62.

091 1.2.9 Silent (missed) miscarriage

A primigravid woman attends the booking clinic at 11 weeks' gestation. An ultrasound examination reveals a silent (missed) miscarriage.

A What are the different management options for this woman? Give two advantages and two disadvantages for each method. (9 marks)

B The woman chooses to have surgery. Discuss this procedure. (7 marks)

C Outline optimal postoperative management. (4 marks)

Key words in the question

- 11 weeks' gestation, miscarriage.
- Different management options.
- Two advantages, two disadvantages, each method.
- Surgery, discuss, procedure.
- Postoperative management.

Essay plan

A

- Expectant management.
- Medical management.
- Surgical management.

B

- ERPC – best option if persistent bleeding, infection, unstable, molar pregnancy or patient's choice.
- Consider cervical priming.
- Vacuum aspiration under general anaesthetic. Oxytocin.
- Complications of ERPC.
- Tissue for histology.

C

- Psychological support, counselling.
- Offer follow-up appointment, support groups.
- Anti-D if rhesus negative.
- Inform GP and community midwife.

Suggested answer

A

There are three options for this woman. They are expectant, medical and surgical management. Expectant management avoids intervention and has a lower incidence of pelvic infection. Disadvantages include that emptying of the uterus takes a longer time and that this method has a lower efficacy (3). The advantages of medical management are that it can be conducted as an out-patient procedure, it avoids a general anaesthetic and the woman has the feeling of being 'more in control'. [It costs £50 less per case to the NHS than surgical treatment.] Disadvantages include an increase in bleeding and pain and that this bleeding may persist for two to three weeks (3). The advantages of surgical evacuation are that the procedure is completed promptly and it is associated with less pain. Possible disadvantages include the need for an anaesthetic and the risk of uterine perforation (3).

B

The procedure is known as evacuation of retained products of conception (ERPC) (1). It is the treatment of choice if there is excessive and persistent bleeding, if the woman is haemodynamically unstable in the presence of infected retained tissue or suspected gestational trophoblastic disease, or (as in this case) if the woman chooses to have surgery (1). Cervical priming may be considered with prostaglandins, as there is evidence that prior to surgical termination of pregnancy prostaglandins reduce the force of dilatation required, haemorrhage, and uterine and cervical trauma (1). The operation is usually performed under general anaesthetic by suction curettage. Vacuum aspiration is preferable to sharp curettage, as it is associated with less pain and blood loss and a shorter operating time (1). Use of routine oxytocin is associated with statistically but not clinically significant reduction in blood loss (1). Complications of ERPC include uterine perforation, cervical tears, intra-abdominal trauma, haemorrhage and intrauterine adhesions (1).

The tissue obtained should be sent for histology to confirm products of conception and to exclude any unsuspected trophoblastic disease (1). [Screening for infections such as chlamydia should be considered and anti-biotics given only if clinically indicated.]

C

She should be provided with psychological support and offered access to formal counselling if necessary. This support may result in significant psychological gain (1). She should be offered a follow-up with the gynaecologist and given information about support groups such as the Miscarriage Association (1). If she is non-sensitized and rhesus negative, she should receive anti-D immunoglobulin within 72 hours of the ERPC (1).

It is essential that all the relevant primary care professionals (particularly her general practitioner and community midwife) be informed of her pregnancy loss (1).

Further reading

Royal College of Obstetricians and Gynaecologists. *The Management of Early Pregnancy Loss*. Green-Top Guideline No. 25. London: RCOG, October 2006.

1.2.10   Cancer of the fallopian tube

Consider a woman presenting with cancer of the fallopian tube.

A   Discuss the predisposing and protective factors. (4 marks)
B   What types of cancer are found in primary disease? (4 marks)
C   What are the presenting symptoms, including the classical presentation, and how is the diagnosis generally made? (4 marks)
D   Outline the FIGO staging of fallopian tube carcinoma. (8 marks)

Key words in the question

- Cancer, fallopian tube.
- Predisposing, protective factors.
- Types, cancer, primary disease.
- Presenting symptoms, classical presentation, diagnosis.
- FIGO staging.

Essay plan

A
- None −? Similar to ovarian cancer, BRCA? COCP and pregnancy protect.

B
- Serous tumours 90%. Mention other types.

C
- Abnormal vaginal bleeding, watery discharge. Classical = hydrops tubae profluens.
- Diagnosis − surgery and histology.

D
- FIGO classification 0−4.

Suggested answer

A

No consistent predisposing factors have been identified. The aetiology may be similar to ovarian carcinoma (1). Structural chromosomal changes including *BRCA1* and *BRCA2* gene mutations have also been implicated in studies (1).

As with ovarian cancer, oral contraceptive use and pregnancy history may significantly decrease tubal cancer risk (2).

B

Serous-type tumours show dominance in primary fallopian tube cancers. More than 90% of fallopian tube carcinomas are papillary serous adenocarcinomas (2).

Other types include endometroid, transitional cell, undifferentiated, clear cell and mixed (2).

C

If there are symptoms, abnormal vaginal bleeding or watery vaginal discharge are the commonest. These may be associated with vague lower abdominal pain, abdominal distension and pressure (2).

The classic description is of hydrops tubae profluens, where a palpable pelvic mass resolves during examination and is associated with watery vaginal discharge (1).

Diagnosis is more frequently made peri- and postoperatively. It is often an incidental finding at laparotomy (1).

D

Fallopian tube cancer is staged by FIGO into stages 0–IV. Stage 0 is carcinoma in situ with no evidence of primary tumour (1).

Stage I is confined to the fallopian tubes. Stage Ia is limited to one tube. Stage Ib is limited to both tubes without penetrating the serosal surfaces. Stage Ic is limited to one or both tubes with extension through the tubal serosa or with ascites or positive washings (2).

Stage II tumour involves one or both fallopian tubes with pelvic extension. In stage IIa the extension is to the uterus and/or ovaries. Stage IIb has extension to other organs. Stage IIc has pelvic extension with positive ascites/washings (2).

Stage III tumour involves one or both fallopian tubes with peritoneal implants outside the pelvis and/or positive lymph nodes. In stage IIIa the metastasis is microscopic. In stage IIIb the metastasis is macroscopic, with the largest dimension being less than 2 cm. In stage IIIc the metastasis is more than 2 cm and/or there are positive regional lymph nodes (2).

Stage IV occurs with distant metastasis beyond the peritoneal cavity (1).

Further reading

Goswami PK, Kerr-Wilson R, McCarthy K. Cancer of the fallopian tube. *The Obstetrician and Gynaecologist* 2006; 8: 147–52.

1.2.11   Endometrial cancer

Mrs Smith is a 64-year-old woman who presents with a solitary episode of postmenopausal bleeding lasting four days.

A   What investigations would you perform to confirm or exclude endometrial cancer? (5 marks)

B   Assuming a diagnosis of endometrial cancer, how can you assess the disease extent before surgery? (5 marks)

C   How is endometrial cancer staged? Describe stage III disease. (6 marks)

D   What are the common indications for post-hysterectomy radiotherapy? (4 marks)

Key words in the question

- Postmenopausal bleeding.
- Investigations, assess, disease extent, before surgery.
- Cancer, staged, describe stage III disease.
- Indications, post-hysterectomy radiotherapy.

Essay plan

A

- TVS and endometrial biopsy, hysteroscopy.

B

- TVS, MRI, CXR.

C

- Surgical staging. Stage III = spread to pelvis.

D

- High-grade tumours, >50% myometrial penetration, positive pelvic lymph nodes, poor histological variants.

Suggested answer

A

A transvaginal ultrasound scan (TVS) should be performed following referral. It is highly reliable for the detection of endometrial cancer (1).

If the endometrial thickness is 5 mm or greater, an endometrial biopsy should be performed. This can be done in the outpatient setting with a device such as a Pipelle aspirator. This can give a correct diagnosis of cancer in over 80% of cases (2).

Diagnostic hysteroscopy and dilatation and curettage should be used when outpatient biopsy is unsuccessful or with persistent abnormal bleeding. This can be undertaken in the outpatient or inpatient setting (2).

B

A TVS and magnetic resonance imaging (MRI) should be used to attempt to assess the endometrial thickness and depth of myometrial invasion. MRI can also look for lymph node involvement and tumour spread beyond the uterus (3).

Tumour grade can be assessed by pathological examination of the biopsy sample (1).

Patients with confirmed disease should have chest radiography to exclude pulmonary metastases (1).

C

Endometrial cancer is staged surgically. Adequate exposure is essential and a midline vertical incision should be used. This allows evaluation of the abdomen, pelvic and para-aortic nodes, and omental biopsy if required (3).

Stage III disease occurs when spread is beyond the uterine body, but not involving the rectal or bladder mucosa and not beyond the abdominal cavity.

It is divided into a, b and c. Stage IIIa involves the serosa of the uterus or adnexae and/or positive cytology. Stage IIIb occurs when there is vaginal involvement, and stage IIIc occurs with involvement of the para-aortic or pelvic lymph node (3).

D

Common indications for post-hysterectomy adjuvant radiotherapy are grades 2 and 3 tumours, myometrial invasion of greater than 50% penetration, cervical involvement, poor histological variants such as clear-cell and papillary serous carcinoma, and positive pelvic lymph nodes (4).

Further reading

Chan YM. Endometrial cancer standards of care. In: Luesley D, Acheson N, eds. *Gynaecological Oncology for the MRCOG and Beyond*. London: RCOG Press, 2004: 109–18.

1.2.12   Hormone replacement therapy

A 49-year-old woman with an intact uterus presents with hot flushes, night sweats and 12 months of amenorrhoea. She requests hormone replacement therapy (HRT).

A How should she be counselled? (10 marks)
B What types of HRT may be suitable for her and why? (5 marks)
C Summarize the non-oestrogen-based treatments available. (5 marks)

Key words in the question

- 49-year-old, hot flushes, amenorrhoea, HRT.
- Counselled.
- Types, HRT.
- Non-oestrogen-based treatments.

Essay plan

A

- Relevant history — gynae, exclude pregnancy.
- Medical, including risk factors osteoporosis.
- Family history DVT, breast and endometrial cancer.
- Benefits v. risks of taking HRT.
- Lifestyle advice.
- Routes of administration.

B

- Continuous combined or cyclical HRT. Unopposed oestrogen contraindicated.

C

- Progestogens alone, clonidine, SSRI/SNRIs, phyto-oestrogens, herbal remedies, homeopathy, acupuncture, reflexology. For prevention osteoporosis consider biphosphonates, SERMs, strontium.

Suggested answer

A

A focused history should be taken, confirming her last menstrual period (LMP), her method of contraception, and whether she has any abnormal bleeding (2).

Risk factors for osteoporosis, e.g. smoking, alcohol, lack of exercise, corticosteroid use and family history of fracture, are enquired about. It is important to ask about family history of deep vein thrombosis (DVT), and breast and endometrial cancer (2).

The patient's history is strongly suggestive of the menopause, although pregnancy should be excluded. The patient should be informed of the benefits of hormone replacement therapy (HRT), including reduction/abolition of hot flushes, reduction in risk of osteoporosis, colon cancer and possibly Alzheimer's disease and an improvement in mood. The risks include an increase in DVT (from 1/10,000 to 3/10,000), a small increase in breast cancer (3 extra cases per 1000 women on HRT for 5 years) and a possible small increase in stroke and cardiovascular disease (4).

The patient should be given lifestyle advice, e.g. to stop smoking and increase exercise if appropriate (1).

The different routes of administration of HRT should be discussed, e.g. oral, transdermal, vaginal or subcutaneous implant (1).

B

HRT is the most beneficial treatment for this woman's vasomotor symptoms. Since she has a uterus, there are two options available. She could have a continuous combined HRT (ccHRT) preparation, consisting of oestrogen and progestogen daily. ccHRT is more popular with postmenopausal women because of the lack of induced bleeding. This patient is suitable for ccHRT, as it is one year since her LMP. She should be advised that irregular bleeding or spotting may occur during the first three to six months of treatment. Patients on ccHRT may have a reduced risk of endometrial cancer compared with cyclical HRT (2).

Alternatively, the patient may be prescribed monthly cyclical or three-monthly cyclical regimes. Both induce a withdrawal bleed, although on the three-monthly regime the patient bleeds only four times a year (2).

A patient with an intact uterus should not be prescribed unopposed oes-trogen due to the marked increase in endometrial hyperplasia and cancer (1).

C

This patient requires treatment for menopausal symptoms. Progestogens, e.g. norethisterone 5 mg daily, may help control hot flushes and night sweats. Clonidine 75 mg b.d. has also been shown to have some benefit in reducing hot flushes. Selective serotonin reuptake inhibitors, e.g. paroxetine and serotonin, and noradrenaline reuptake inhibitors, e.g. venlafaxine, are effective in treating hot flushes in the short term (3).

Phyto-oestrogens, e.g. isoflavones, herbal remedies, e.g. ginseng or black cohosh, homeopathy, acupuncture and reflexology have all been widely used to treat menopausal symptoms. Unfortunately, there is no good evidence that any of these complementary or alternative therapies work (1).

If HRT is contraindicated or declined, agents such as biphosphonates, selective oestrogen receptor modulators or strontium ranelate are useful in the prevention of osteoporosis but will not help her vasomotor symptoms (1).

Further reading

Rees M. *Menopause for the MRCOG and Beyond.* London: RCOG Press, 2008.
Rees M, Purdie DW, eds. *Management of the Menopause: The Handbook* (4th edition). London: RSM Press, 2006.

1.2.13 Subfertility

A 32-year-old woman attends the fertility clinic with her partner. They have a two-year history of subfertility.

A What aspects of the history and examination should be ascertained at this consultation? (13 marks)
B What investigations may be useful in order to establish the cause of their subfertility? (4 marks)
C What lifestyle advice should be given to this couple to enhance their chances of conception? (3 marks)

Key words in the question

- 32-year-old, two-year history, subfertility.
- History, examination.
- Investigations, establish, cause, subfertility.
- Lifestyle advice, enhance, conception.

Essay plan

A
- Ask questions relating to subfertility, medical, surgical, sexual and occupational.
- General exam, male and female genital.

B
- Sperm.
- Blood tests.
- Tubal patency.

C
- Smoking, alcohol and weight.

Suggested answer

A

I would ask the couple questions relating to their infertility, medical and surgical history, and sexual and occupational history. Relevant points in the infertility history are pregnancy in the current and/or previous relationships

(1). It is important to establish the length and type of previous contraceptive use and whether either of the couple has had previous investigations or treatment for infertility (2). Additional medical information required from the woman is her menstrual history, including cycle length, regularity, dysmenorrhoea and menorrhagia (1). Both partners should be asked about sexually transmitted infections, particularly epididymitis and pelvic inflammatory disease (PID) (1), and alcohol, smoking, substance misuse and chronic disease (1). In the male, a history of mumps and maldescent of the testes should be asked about (1).

Surgical history should cover any abdominal or pelvic surgery in the woman and testicular or hernia surgery in the man (1). Occupational history should include any exposure to toxic substances and any significant time spent away from home as a consequence of work (1). Sexual history should establish the frequency and timing of intercourse, and coital habits. Sensitive enquiry is made to exclude premature ejaculation, lack of libido and impotence (1).

General examination of both partners should include body mass index (BMI), blood pressure, and fat and hair distribution (check for hirsutism in the woman) (1). In the male, the inguinal canal and genitalia should be examined and any abnormality noted (1). In the female an abdominal and pelvic examination should be performed and any abnormality recorded (1).

B

Semen analysis should be performed and if the first result is abnormal, this must be repeated after one to three months (1).

In a regular menstrual cycle, the luteal phase progesterone (collected on day 21 in a 28-day cycle) should confirm ovulation (1). In cases of oligomenorrhoea or amenorrhoea, follicle-stimulating hormone, luteinizing hormone, prolactin, testosterone and serum hormone-binding globulin should be measured in an attempt to ascertain the cause of anovulation (1).

Tubal patency should be assessed. This can be done using a hysterosalpingogram, hysterosalpingo-contrast-ultrasonography (HyCosy), or a laparoscopy and dye test (1).

[The woman's rubella status should be established before she tries further to become pregnant. If she is not immune, she can be immunized and advised to avoid pregnancy for at least a month after immunization. This is not a test for infertility so it is irrelevant to this part of the question.]

C

If either of the couple smokes, they should be advised to stop (1). Alcohol intake should be limited to one or two units once or twice a week for the woman, while men should keep to the Department of Health's recommendation of a maximum four units per day (1). If either of the couple has a BMI >30 kg/m^2, they should be advised to lose weight. Women with a BMI of <19 kg/m^2 should be advised to gain weight (1).

Further reading

Hamilton M. The initial assessment of the infertile couple. In: Bhattacharya S, Hamilton M, eds. *Management of Infertility for the MRCOG and Beyond* (2nd edition). London: RCOG Press, 2007: 11–21.

National Institute for Health and Clinical Excellence. *Fertility: Assessment and Treatment for People with Fertility Problems.* Clinical Guideline No. 11. London: NICE, February 2004.

1.2.14   Vulval cancer

A Discuss the incidence, age group affected and predisposing factors associated with vulval cancer. What is the commonest type of tumour? (5 marks)

B Outline the FIGO staging of this disease. (7 marks)

C How would you treat a stage Ia tumour? (2 marks)

D What are the complications associated with vulval and inguinal surgery? (6 marks)

Key words in the question

- Predisposing factors, vulval cancer.
- FIGO staging.
- Treat, stage Ia.
- Complications, vulval and inguinal surgery.

Essay plan

A

- Aetiological factors associated with vulval cancer and commonest type.

B

- FIGO classification 0, Ia, Ib, II, III, IVa, IVb.

C

- Describe treatment of Ia tumours.

D

- Complications of vulval and inguinal surgery.

Suggested answer

A

Vulval cancer is rare. Its incidence is approximately 1.7/100,000 women. It is a disease that affects women predominantly in their 70s and 80s. Predisposing factors for developing vulval cancer include lichen sclerosus, vulval intra-epithelial neoplasia (VIN), Paget's disease and melanoma in situ. Ninety per cent of these tumours are squamous cell carcinomas (5).

B

Vulval cancer is classified by FIGO into stage 0, Ia, Ib, II, III, IVa or IVb.

Stage 0 is carcinoma in situ or preinvasive cancer (1).

In stage I disease the tumour is confined to the vulva or vulva and perineum with the greatest dimension being 2 cm or less. In stage Ia the stromal invasion is no greater than 1 mm. In stage Ib disease the stromal invasion is greater than 1 mm (2).

In stage II the tumour is still confined to the vulva or vulva and perineum but is more than 2 cm in its greatest dimension (1).

In stage III disease the tumour invades the lower urethra, vagina or anus and/or there is unilateral regional lymph node metastasis (1).

In stage IVa the tumour invades any of the following: bladder mucosa, rectal mucosa, upper urethral mucosa, bilateral regional nodes and bone (1).

Stage IVb occurs with distant metastasis, including pelvic lymph nodes (1).

C

The treatment of vulval cancer is primarily surgical. In stage Ia disease the treatment is by wide excision only, with no groin node dissection, as the risk of lymph node involvement is negligible. A minimum margin of 15 mm of disease-free tissue is recommended (2).

D

The complications associated with vulval and inguinal surgery include wound breakdown and infection, thromboembolism, urinary incontinence, inguinal lymphocyst, lymphoedema, introital stenosis and psychosexual problems (6).

Further reading

Royal College of Obstetricians and Gynaecologists. *The Management of Vulval Cancer*. Working Party Report. London: RCOG, January 2006.

1.2.15 Laparoscopy

You have decided to perform diagnostic laparoscopy for pelvic pain.

A What are the relevant points that should be discussed at the time of taking consent? (Do not include anaesthetic complications.) (11 marks)

B Discuss a safe closed-entry laparoscopic technique. (9 marks)

Key words in the question

- Diagnostic laparoscopy, pelvic pain.
- Relevant, discussed, consent.
- Discuss, safe closed-entry, laparoscopic technique.

Essay plan

A

- Explain and confirm need for surgery.
- Explain all risks from surgery, with their incidence.

B

- Open- v. closed-entry technique.
- Safe insertion of Verres needle.
- Correct intra-abdominal pressures.

Suggested answer

A

Comprehensive consent is essential for diagnostic laparoscopy, as it is associated with serious complications in 1 in 1000 cases (1). A detailed history and examination should confirm that laparoscopy is appropriate, and this should be documented. The procedure must be explained to the patient and all risks and complications discussed (1). Most complications arise from insertion of the Verres needle or the entry trocar (1). This can cause injury to the bowel, bladder or blood vessels (1). The incidence varies greatly depending on operator experience and the complexity of the case, in particular with extremes of BMI, previous abdominal surgery or previous inflammatory bowel disease. The incidence of these complications varies between 1 and 12.5/1000 (2). Bowel injury is more common than vessel injury (1). Unfortunately, not all bowel injuries are noticed at the time of the operation – some become manifest only after discharge home. Patients must be warned of this possibility (1). If the injury is serious, it may require reparative surgery at the time or later (1). The entry wounds may become infected and a later complication of the entry sites is hernia formation (1). The patient may experience shoulder tip pain for 24–48 hours after the operation from gas trapped under the diaphragm (1).

B

A safe entry begins with the correct positioning of the operating table. The table should initially be horizontal and should be changed to the Trendelenburg position (head-down tilt) only after the trocars have been inserted (1). A vertical incision of the skin should be made, starting from the umbilicus downwards, avoiding entry into the peritoneal cavity (1). The Verres needle used should be sharp and have a good spring action to decrease the risk of injury due to excessive force. A disposable needle is preferable (1). The lower abdominal wall should be stabilized in such a way that the Verres needle is inserted at right angles to the skin, thus decreasing the length traversed by the needle before it enters the peritoneal cavity (1). If two attempts at umbilical Verres needle insertion have failed to gain access to the peritoneal cavity, an open laparoscopy (Hasson's technique) or insertion of the Verres needle at Palmer's point should be performed (1). When inside the peritoneal cavity, excessive lateral movement of the Verres needle must not be performed, as that can exacerbate any visceral injury (1). The initial insufflation pressure should be under 8 mmHg (1). The intra-abdominal pressure should be 20–25 mmHg before the insertion of the trocars. This pressure gives adequate splinting of the anterior abdominal wall, permitting safe entry (1). A 360° examination around the entry site must be carried out before proceeding to check for any injury (1).

Further reading

Royal College of Obstetricians and Gynaecologists. *Preventing Entry-Related Gynaecological Laparoscopic Injuries*. Green-Top Guideline No. 49. London: RCOG, May 2008.

1.2.16 Overactive bladder syndrome

A 62-year-old woman attends your gynaecology clinic with symptoms of overactive bladder syndrome (OABS).

A Outline the characteristics associated with OABS. (4 marks)

B Discuss the treatments that may be offered to this patient, assuming the diagnosis of OABS. (10 marks)

C What are the main complications associated with the surgical treatment of OABS? (6 marks)

Key words in the question

- Overactive bladder syndrome (OABS).
- Characteristics.
- Treatments.
- Complications, surgical treatment.

Essay plan

A

- Define OABS and its associated characteristics, including urge incontinence or its absence.

B

- Outline the conservative therapies, drug therapies and surgical management.

C

- Complications of sacral nerve stimulation, botulinum toxin A injected in the bladder, augmentation cystoplasty and urinary diversion.

Suggested answer

A

Overactive bladder syndrome (OABS) is defined as urgency that occurs with or without urge incontinence and usually with frequency (greater than eight voids per day) and nocturia. This occurs in the absence of another identifiable process affecting the lower urinary tract. OABS that occurs with urge incontinence is known as OABS 'wet', while that without is known as OABS 'dry' (4).

B

OABS can be treated by conservative therapies, drug therapies and surgical management (1).

Conservative therapies include lifestyle interventions such as reducing tea/coffee intake, modification of fluid intake to approximately 1.5–2 litres fluid per day and, in those women with a body mass index (BMI) of greater than 30 kg/m^2, weight reduction (2).

Bladder training lasting a minimum of six weeks should be commenced, preferably via a continence adviser, to increase the times between voids and increase bladder capacity (2).

Should these measures prove ineffective, an anticholinergic preparation can be prescribed. The National Institute for Health and Clinical Excellence (NICE) recommends immediate-release oxybutinin 5 mg three times daily as first-line therapy. If this does not help or is not tolerated, then another anticholinergic such as tolterodine, solifenacin or trospium can be prescribed. These may be long-acting. Transdermal preparations of oxybutinin may also be tried (2).

Intravaginal oestrogens can be tried in those postmenopausal women with vaginal atrophy (1).

Surgery can be offered to those patients in whom medical treatment fails. Procedures include sacral nerve stimulation, botulinum toxin A injected in the bladder, augmentation cystoplasty and urinary diversion (2).

C

Complications of sacral nerve stimulation include failure and the need to reoperate (1). Complications of botulinum toxin A include failure and the need to self-catheterize; also, injections have to be repeated every nine months to one year (2). Complications of augmentation cystoplasty include bowel disturbance, metabolic acidosis, the need to self-catheterize, mucus retention and malignant change (2). Complications of urinary diversion include bowel disturbance and stoma herniation and retraction (1).

Further reading

Munjuluri N, Wong W, Yoong W. Anticholinergic drugs for overactive bladder: a review of the literature and practical guide. *The Obstetrician and Gynaecologist* 2007; 9: 9–14.

National Institute for Health and Clinical Excellence. *The Management of Urinary Incontinence in Women.* NICE Clinical Guideline No. 40. London: NICE, October 2006.

1.2.17 Polycystic ovarian syndrome

A 31-year-old woman attends the gynaecological outpatient clinic with a three-year history of oligomenorrhoea and hirsutism. Her body mass index (BMI) is 38 kg/m^2. You suspect she has polycystic ovarian syndrome (PCOS).

A How would you confirm the diagnosis of PCOS? (5 marks)

B Assuming the diagnosis is PCOS, how would you counsel this patient? (15 marks)

Key words in the question

- 31-year-old, three-year history, oligomenorrhoea, hirsutism, BMI 38 kg/m^2.
- Confirm, PCOS.
- Counsel, patient.

Essay plan

A

- Exclude other diseases – baseline investigations.
- Must have 2 of 3 criteria.

B

- Lifestyle factors.
- Discuss long-term risks.

Suggested answer

A

The diagnosis is made by excluding other diseases such as hyperprolactinae-mia, congenital adrenal hyperplasia, androgen-secreting tumours, thyroid disorders and Cushing syndrome. Recommended tests are thyroid function, serum prolactin and free androgen index (1). If total testosterone is >5 nmol/l, 17-hydroxyprogesterone should be measured (1). The diagnosis of polycystic ovarian syndrome (PCOS) can be made if two of the three following criteria are present: polycystic ovaries (12 or more peripheral follicles or increased ovarian volume >10 cm³ on ultrasound scan) (1); oligo- or anovulation (1); clinical and/or biochemical signs of hyperandrogenism (1).

B

This patient should be counselled about the long-term risks to her health and advised to lose weight and increase exercise in order to achieve a BMI of 20–25 kg/m² (2). This patient is at an increased risk of type II diabetes, as her BMI is 38 kg/m². She requires a glucose tolerance test and annual screening for diabetes (1).

Other long-term risks include sleep apnoea, cardiovascular risk factors, implications if she becomes pregnant, and increased risk of endometrial hyperplasia and cancer. She should be asked about snoring and daytime tiredness and offered investigation and treatment if she has sleep apnoea (1).

This woman is significantly overweight. Cardiovascular risk factors include hypertension, obesity, hyperandrogenism, hyperlipidaemia and hyperinsulinaemia. Elevation of some of these factors may put this patient at an increased risk of accelerated atherosclerosis, which may result in myocardial infarction. Should her blood pressure persistently be >140/90 mmHg, she should be commenced on antihypertensives. Statins are not recommended routinely but may be prescribed by a specialist (5).

If this patient becomes pregnant, she should be screened for gestational diabetes before 20 weeks and referral to obstetric diabetic clinic arranged if abnormal. Metformin is neither recommended nor licensed in pregnancy (3). Should this woman have oligo- or amenorrhoea, she is at an increased risk of endometrial hyperplasia and eventually carcinoma. She should have a regular induction of a withdrawal bleed, e.g. with an oral contraceptive pill, cyclical progestogens or Mirena (3).

Further reading

Royal College of Obstetricians and Gynaecologists. *Long-Term Consequences of Polycystic Ovary Syndrome*. Green-Top Guideline No. 33. London: RCOG, December 2007.

1.2.18 Complications of postvaginal hysterectomy

You are the registrar on call and you are asked to see a 66-year-old, well-controlled hypertensive woman who has had a vaginal hysterectomy with pelvic floor repair four hours ago. She has a blood pressure of 70/50 mmHg and pulse of 138 beats per minute.

A What features would you look for on clinical examination? (6 marks)

B What is the likely diagnosis? (1 mark)

C Justify your investigations. (3 marks)

D Outline your further management. (10 marks)

Key words in the question

- 66-year-old, vaginal hysterectomy, pelvic floor repair four hours ago.
- Blood pressure, 70/50 mmHg, pulse, 138 beats per minute.
- Features, clinical examination.
- Likely diagnosis.
- Investigations.
- Outline, management.

Essay plan

A

- Evidence of hypovolaemia, review postoperative vital sign chart and operation notes.
- Examine abdomen, vagina, chest.

B

- Haemorrhage.

C

- FBC, clotting screen and cross-match.

D

- Resuscitation – ABC.
- Inform anaesthetist, consultant gynae, theatre.
- Vaginal approach, if unsuccessful laparotomy.
- Suture bleeding points, continue resuscitation.
- HDU or ITU if necessary.
- Full explanation to patient.

Suggested answer

A

I would look for other evidence of hypovolaemia – cold, pale, sweaty, cyanosed skin with delayed capillary refill, alteration of her mental state (e.g. confusion, reduced consciousness), a fall in her hourly urine output since surgery (due to reduced perfusion), and a narrowed pulse pressure (due to increased diastolic blood pressure reflecting vasoconstriction) (2). The increased heart rate is an early sign of compensation in hypovolaemic shock, while a reduction in blood pressure is usually a late sign. I would review her postoperative vital sign chart of previous hourly pulse rate and blood pressure to note whether there has been a steady decline in pressure and rise in pulse rate. Patients often lose 30–40% (1.5–2 litres) of their circulating blood volume before the systolic blood pressure falls (1). I would also review the operation notes to identify any difficulty the surgeon may have had during the vaginal hysterectomy (1).

I would examine the abdomen for signs of intra-abdominal haemorrhage – distension, guarding and rigidity. Some or all of these signs will be present if she has a significant intraperitoneal bleed (1). I would examine her chest for crepitations and diminished air entry. Vaginal examination may reveal per vaginal loss (1).

B

The most likely diagnosis is hypovolaemia secondary to haemorrhage (1).

C

Appropriate investigations include urgent full blood count (for haemoglobin and platelet estimation) (1) and clotting screen (to detect coagulopathy) (1); six units of blood should be cross-matched with the proviso that more may be required (1).

D

Since this patient is very likely to have non-compressible haemorrhage, I would commence resuscitation following the ABC principle – oxygen at 15 litres/minute via a tight-fitting face-mask and restoration of adequate circulating volume until the bleeding can be arrested (1). Two large-bore cannulas should be sited and the patient commenced on crystalloids and later colloids (all fluids require warming to avoid hypothermia) (1). I would inform theatres and my anaesthetic on-call colleague and ask him/her to review the patient with a view to return to theatre for examination under anaesthetic and possibly a laparotomy. I would inform the on-call consultant gynaecologist and ask him/her to attend (1). Under general anaesthetic the vaginal sutures can be undone and if a pedicle is bleeding, this can be ligated (1). If it is not possible to identify the source of the bleeding, or the patient continues to haemorrhage, laparotomy should be performed (1). The source of the bleeding should be isolated and occluded with tissue forceps or compression and gently sutured under direct vision (1). During this time the anaesthetist will continue resuscitation, including transfusing the patient with blood and fresh frozen plasma or other blood products, being guided by the patient's clotting screen and haemoglobin values and often supported by advice from a haematologist (1). On request, the anaesthetist will return the patient's blood pressure to normal, and the peritoneal cavity should be inspected for further bleeding before the abdomen is closed. After ensuring of haemostasis, a drain may be inserted to allow any residual ooze to escape (1). Depending on her condition she may require high-dependency care or intensive care for 24–48 hours (1).

As soon as possible following surgery the patient should be given a thorough explanation of the events and likely consequences (if any) of the complication (1). [An incident form should be completed and the case reviewed by the risk management team and any lessons learnt disseminated.]

Further reading

Grady K. Shock. In: Grady K, Howell C, Cox C, eds. *Managing Obstetric Emergencies and Trauma. The MOET Course Manual* (2nd edition). London: RCOG, 2007: 97–106.

Oram D. The abdominal approach to pelvic surgery. In: Maxwell DJ, ed. *Surgical Techniques in Obstetrics and Gynaecology.* London: Churchill Livingstone, 2004: 97–109.

1.2.19   Acute pelvic inflammatory disease

A 19-year-old girl is referred with a three-day history of lower abdominal pain and tenderness and offensive vaginal discharge. She has been sexually active with her current partner for one month.

A   What other features would suggest a diagnosis of acute pelvic inflammatory disease (PID)? (3 marks)

B   If the diagnosis was uncertain, what three investigations would be the most helpful? (3 marks)

C   Assuming moderate PID is confirmed, outline a suitable management plan. (7 marks)

D   When should patients with acute PID be admitted to hospital? (3 marks)

E   When should surgical treatment be considered? Mention three possible methods. (4 marks)

Key words in the question

- 19-year-old, three-day history, lower abdominal pain, tenderness, offensive vaginal discharge.
- Sexually active, current partner, one month.
- Features, acute PID.
- Three investigations.
- Suitable management plan.
- When, admitted to hospital.
- Surgical treatment, three possible methods.

Essay plan

A

- Deep dyspareunia, cervical excitation, fever.

B

- Endocervical swabs, laparoscopy, transvaginal ultrasound.

C

- Treat as outpatient.
- Ofloxacin and metronidazole.
- Written information and long-term implications.
- Contact tracing.

D

- Lack of response or intolerant to oral therapy.
- If a surgical emergency not excluded.
- Tubo-ovarian abscess.
- Clinically severe disease.

E

- Pelvic abscess, tubo-ovarian mass.
- Three methods: ultrasound drainage, laparoscopy, laparotomy.

Suggested answer

A

Other features associated with acute pelvic inflammatory disease (PID) are deep dyspareunia, cervical excitation and adnexal tenderness, and a temperature above 38 °C (3).

B

Three helpful investigations are endocervical swabs for chlamydia and gonorrhoea, diagnostic laparoscopy and transvaginal ultrasound (3).

C

This patient can be treated as an outpatient (1). A suitable regime is oral ofloxacin 400 mg b.d. and oral metronidazole 400 mg b.d. for 14 days (2). The woman should be informed about the diagnosis and the potential long-term implications for her health (1). She should be given written information about PID (1). She should be advised to visit the genitourinary medicine clinic with her partner to facilitate contact tracing and infection screening (2).

D

Admission to hospital is appropriate if the patient fails to respond to or is intolerant of oral therapy, if a surgical emergency cannot be excluded, if a tubo-ovarian abscess is present, or if the patient has clinically severe disease (3).

E

Surgical intervention should be considered in severe cases or where a pelvic abscess or tubo-ovarian mass is present (1). Methods of surgical treatment include ultrasound drainage, laparoscopic drainage and laparotomy with drainage (3).

Further reading

Royal College of Obstetricians and Gynaecologists. *Management of Acute Pelvic Inflammatory Disease*. Green-Top Guideline No. 32. London: RCOG, May 2003.

1.2.20   Postmenopausal ovarian cyst

A 63-year-old postmenopausal woman is referred to the gynaecological clinic by her general practitioner with an ovarian cyst 5 cm in diameter apparent on transabdominal ultrasound scan.

A What investigations are appropriate in this case and why? (6 marks)

B If results of these investigations suggest that the patient has a very low risk (<3%) of having ovarian cancer, outline your management. (9 marks)

C If investigations reveal a high risk of ovarian cancer, how should she be managed? (5 marks)

Key words in the question

- Postmenopausal woman, ovarian cyst, 5 cm, transabdominal ultrasound.
- Investigations.
- Very low risk, ovarian cancer, outline, management.
- High risk, ovarian cancer, managed.

Essay plan

A

- CA125, transvaginal ultrasound scan, calculate risk of malignancy index.

B

- Conservative management, woman's opinion.

C

- Surgical management in cancer centre, laparotomy. Cytology, biopsies of suspicious areas, TAH/BSO + omentectomy.

Suggested answer

A

Appropriate investigations in this case include determining the cancer antigen 125 (CA125) level and transvaginal ultrasound scan (TVS), as this information enables triaging of the patient in deciding the most appropriate place for her to be managed. CA125 is raised in over 80% of ovarian cancers, and using a cut-off of 30 U/ml the test has a sensitivity of 81% and specificity of 75%. TVS is more sensitive than transabdominal ultrasound (4).

The 'risk of malignancy index' should be calculated. This value enables the gynaecologist to decide whether this woman requires surgery in a cancer centre by a gynaecological oncologist or whether a general gynaecologist can manage her. The 'risk of malignancy index' (RMI) is calculated as follows:

$$RMI = U \times M \times CA125$$

where U = ultrasound score, $M = 3$ for all postmenopausal women and CA125 is serum CA125 measurement in U/ml (2).

B

Since the risk of ovarian cancer is very low, this patient can be managed conservatively by a general gynaecologist (1).

Her RMI is likely to be <25 since she has <3% risk of ovarian cancer. Many of these cysts will resolve spontaneously within three months (1).

Prudent management entails repeat TVS and serum CA125 every four months for a year (2).

If the cyst resolves or there is no change in it after one year (three scans), the patient can be safely discharged from follow-up (2).

Aspiration is not recommended in the management of ovarian cysts in postmenopausal women, as cytological examination is poor at distinguishing between benign and malignant tumours (1).

If the woman requests surgery, then laparoscopic oophorectomy is appropriate; if that is unavailable, open oophorectomy may be undertaken (2).

C

Since the risk of ovarian cancer is high, she requires surgical intervention by a gynaecological oncologist in a cancer centre (1).

She will likely have a RMI of >250. The gynaecological oncologist will perform a staging laparotomy through an extended midline incision, including cytology of ascites or washings, total abdominal hysterectomy and bilateral salpingo-oophorectomy (BSO), and infra-colic omentectomy and biopsies from suspicious areas (3).

She may require postoperative chemotherapy, depending on the stage of her cancer (1).

Further reading

Royal College of Obstetricians and Gynaecologists. *Ovarian Cysts in Postmenopausal Women*. Green-Top Guideline No. 34. London: RCOG, October 2003.

1.2.21 Emergency contraception and laparoscopic clip sterilization

A Identify two methods of emergency contraception. When would you prescribe it and what advice would you give to a patient receiving emergency contraception? (13 marks)

B What factors are important in counselling a woman in the outpatient clinic requesting laparoscopic clip sterilization? Do not discuss specific risks associated with laparoscopy. (7 marks)

Key words in the question

- Two methods, emergency contraception.
- When, prescribe, what advice.
- Factors, important, counselling, sterilization.

Essay plan

A

- Progestogen only and CuIUD.
- Unprotected intercourse, condom accident.
- Levonorgestrel – within 72 hours, vomiting, advice re next period.
- CuIUD more effective and up to 5 days.
- STI screen and antibiotic prophylaxis.
- Enzyme inducers.

B

- Offer long-acting reversible contraception – advantages, disadvantages, failure rate and leaflets. Mention vasectomy.
- Permanent – reversal unlikely on NHS. Failure rate, ectopic possibility.
- Continue current method contraception until next period.

Suggested answer

A

Two effective methods of emergency contraception (EC) are oral progestogen-only levonorgestrel and the copper intrauterine device (IUD) (1).

EC is given after unprotected intercourse or condom accident. It may also be given if the woman has sexual intercourse after she misses/forgets to take the combined pill during the first week of her cycle (1).

I would explain to the patient that the tablet (levonorgestrel 1.5 mg) is effective if taken within 72 hours of unprotected intercourse, and the sooner it is taken following intercourse the more likely it is to work (1). Should vomiting occur within three hours of taking the tablet, a further dose can be given (1). I would also inform the patient that her next period might be early or late (1). She should use a barrier method of contraception, e.g. condom, until her next period, to reduce the likelihood of pregnancy (1). If she develops any lower abdominal pain, she should seek urgent assessment to exclude ectopic pregnancy (1). If she subsequently (in the next three or four weeks) has a menstrual bleed that is abnormally light, brief, heavy or absent, she should also seek medical advice (1).

I would explain to the woman that the copper IUD is more effective than the hormonal tablet method, although it does require a small procedure to insert it (1). It can be inserted up to five days after unprotected intercourse (1). Sexually transmitted diseases should be tested for and insertion of the IUD covered by antibiotic prophylaxis (1). Should intercourse have occurred more than five days previously, the IUD can still be used provided that the earliest likely calculated ovulation date is within five days of insertion (1). If this patient is on an enzyme-inducing medication, I would advise her to have the IUD inserted or to take two doses of levonorgestrel 1.5 mg 12 hours apart.

This is because the standard dose may be ineffective, owing to increased metabolism. The increased dose is not currently licensed (1).

B

It is important to provide information to women about other long-term reversible methods of contraception, e.g. Mirena, Implanon, Depo-Provera and copper intrauterine devices. This should include the advantages, disadvantages and relative failure rates of each method (1). Verbal counselling should be supported by accurate leaflets and information that the woman can take away and read prior to surgery (1). The patient should be informed that if her partner opts for a vasectomy, that procedure has a lower failure rate (1 in 2000), has less morbidity and can be performed under local anaesthetic (1).

She should be informed that sterilization is intended to be permanent, but she should be given information about the success rates of reversal. However, women need to be aware that it is very unlikely that the NHS will fund reversal operations (1).

The patient needs to know the lifetime failure rate with female sterilization is estimated to be 1 in 200. Most laparoscopic clip sterilizations (LCSs) in the UK use Filshie® clips, and the failure rate with these clips after 10 years is 2–3/1000 (1). Women should be informed that if LCS fails, the resulting pregnancy may be ectopic. If they think they might be pregnant, they should seek medical advice early (1). The patient should be advised to continue with her current method of contraception, e.g. condoms or combined pill, until her next menstrual period after the sterilization (1). [If sterilization is requested postpartum or post-termination, the patient should be informed of the increased regret rate and possibly an increased failure rate. The RCOG recommends that if tubal occlusion is to be performed at the same time as caesarean section, counselling agreement should have been obtained at least one week prior to surgery.]

Further reading

Brechin S, Bigrigg A. Male and female sterilisation. *Current Obstetrics and Gynaecology* 2006; **16**: 39–46.

Emergency contraception, section 7.3.5. *British National Formulary* (BNF), No. 52, March 2008: 437–8.

Royal College of Obstetricians and Gynaecologists. *Male and Female Sterilisation*. Evidence-Based Clinical Guideline No. 4. London: RCOG, January 2004.

1.2.22 Stress urinary incontinence

A 45-year-old woman with a body mass index (BMI) of 35 kg/m^2 presents to the gynaecology clinic with symptoms suggestive of stress urinary incontinence (SUI). She has had no treatment from her general practitioner.

A What information would help you to make a diagnosis of 'pure' stress incontinence? (12 marks)

B Assuming a diagnosis of 'pure' stress incontinence in this case, what would be your immediate management plan (non-surgical)? Explain why and how and over what timescale it would be given. (8 marks)

Key words in the question

- 45-year-old, BMI of 35 kg/m^2, SUI, no treatment.
- Information, diagnosis, 'pure' stress incontinence.
- 'Pure' stress incontinence, immediate management plan, non-surgical, why, how, timescale.

Essay plan

A

- History, examination and investigation in the OPD.

B

- Outline conservative therapy including lifestyle changes, physiotherapy and drugs, *not* surgery.

Suggested answer

A

In any clinical situation it is important that a detailed and accurate history is taken (1). In this case, it is important to elicit when the patient is incontinent and while doing what activities. In 'pure' stress incontinence the patients leak urine when raised abdominal pressure is higher than urethral closure pressure. This can occur with coughing, laughing, sneezing and physical activity (2).

There should be no history of symptoms of overactive bladder, including urgency, urge incontinence, frequency and nocturia (2).

There should no symptoms of voiding dysfunction, such as hesitancy, poor stream, double voiding, incomplete emptying or terminal dribbling (1).

A three-day urinary diary will help to ascertain this information (1).

Examination of the patient is performed to exclude urinary retention, pelvic mass and prolapse, although this can be present in 'pure' stress incontinence to some degree. Leakage should be seen when the patient is examined in the left lateral position with a comfortably full bladder when intra-abdominal pressure is raised, e.g. coughing (2).

An assessment of her pelvic floor muscle contraction should be undertaken by digital examination (1).

The urine should be dipsticked to detect the presence of blood, glucose, protein and nitrites. If these tests are negative, there is no need to obtain a mid-stream specimen of urine (1).

She does not need urodynamics at this stage (1).

B

As this patient has had no therapy, the first-line treatment would be conservative (1). This involves lifestyle advice such as weight loss (1).

The patient should be referred to a physiotherapist trained in pelvic floor function for a trial of supervised pelvic floor muscle training lasting at least three months. It is important that these women are appropriately supervised, as it has been shown that up to 50% of women cannot perform pelvic floor exercises correctly. When the exercises are supervised appropriately, improvement is seen in up to 40–60%. The women should undertake eight contractions of their pelvic floor three times a day as a minimum. If they cannot contract their pelvic floor well, then electrical stimulation and/or biofeedback should be considered (5).

There is currently only one pharmacological agent available for stress urinary incontinence, namely duloxetine. However, it is not currently recommended by the National Institute for Health and Clinical Excellence for first-line treatment (1).

Further reading

Johnson H, Slack M. Evidence-based management of stress urinary incontinence. *The Obstetrician and Gynaecologist* 2005; 7: 159–65.
National Institute for Health and Clinical Excellence. *The Management of Urinary Incontinence in Women.* Clinical Guideline No. 40. London: NICE, October 2006.

1.2.23   Cervical cancer

A patient is referred to the gynaecology clinic with possible cervical cancer.

A   Where should this patient be seen? What findings would raise the index of suspicion of cervical cancer? How would you confirm the diagnosis? (5 marks)

B   The diagnosis is confirmed as stage Ib cervical cancer. What is stage Ib cervical cancer? Discuss the options for treatment in this situation. (11 marks)

C   What post-treatment support and follow-up are required? (4 marks)

Key words in the question

- Possible cervical cancer.
- Where, seen, findings, raise, index of suspicion, confirm, diagnosis.
- Stage Ib, options, treatment.
- Post-treatment, follow-up.

Essay plan

- Colposcopy. Large, irregular cervix, increased vascularity. Biopsy.
- Stage Ib = confined to cervix. Surgery and radiotherapy equally effective. Retain fertility or not.
- Usually five years. Potential physical, psychological and sexual morbidity, counselling.

Suggested answer

A

A woman with clinically suspected cervical cancer is best seen in a colposcopy clinic (1).

At colposcopy the presence of a large lesion, abnormal blood vessels or an irregular surface contour would raise the index of suspicion (2).

If invasive disease is suspected, then a biopsy is obtained. If small, this could include the whole lesion. If large, then a biopsy is sufficient, as attempting to remove the entire lesion tends not to enhance diagnostic accuracy and can cause complications (2).

B

In stage Ib cervical cancer, the lesion is confined to the cervix. It can be subdivided into stage Ib1, where the lesion is 4 cm or less in diameter, and stage Ib2, where it is greater than 4 cm (2).

The currently available evidence suggests that stage Ib tumours are equally effectively treated by surgery and radiotherapy (1).

In small stage Ib1 tumours, fertility may be retained. The patient can be offered lymphadenectomy and trachelectomy (2).

For those patients who do not wish to retain their fertility, the options are either radical hysterectomy with lymphadenectomy or radical radiotherapy. Surgery should be undertaken by a specialist gynaecological oncologist working in a cancer centre, as this increases the five-year survival rate. Surgery should be offered where possible since it is less likely to result in impairment of bowel or bladder function and sexual enjoyment (2).

Radical radiotherapy should be used in those patients who opt for it, in those who are unfit for surgery, where the surgery is unlikely to remove the tumour completely, or where the risk of requiring postoperative radiotherapy is considered high. This should reduce the likelihood of patients receiving both surgery and radiotherapy, as this has been shown to be associated with a higher morbidity (2).

A clinical oncologist with a gynaecological interest is best suited to deliver this treatment. It should consist of radiotherapy and chemoradiation, and is usually given in the form of intracavity brachytherapy and external beam radiotherapy (2).

C

There is no reliable evidence regarding follow-up of patients with cervical cancer. Most cancer centres follow up patients for five years and then discharge if all is well. There is no evidence to support the use of cytology (2).

Treatment of these cancers can result in physical, psychosocial and sexual morbidity. Patients should receive help, support and counselling in these areas. Clear routes for access to specialist services should be available if patients develop other specific problems such as lymphoedema, and bowel and bladder problems (2).

Further reading

Acheson N. Presentation, investigation and diagnosis. In: Luesley D, Acheson N, eds. *Gynaecological Oncology for the MRCOG and Beyond*. London: RCOG Press, 2004: 45–52.

Mann C, Luesley D. Cervical cancer standards of care. In: Luesley D, Acheson N, eds. *Gynaecological Oncology for the MRCOG and Beyond*. London: RCOG Press, 2004: 119–30.

1.2.24 Ovarian hyperstimulation syndrome

A 36-year-old woman undergoing in vitro fertilization (IVF) treatment is admitted with severe abdominal pain and vomiting.

A Excluding ovarian hyperstimulation syndrome (OHSS), what differential diagnoses should be considered in this woman? (3 marks)

B Discuss how OHSS is classified. (9 marks)

C In this case justify your examination and any investigations you may wish to perform. (8 marks)

Key words in the question

- IVF treatment.
- Severe abdominal pain, vomiting.
- Excluding OHSS, differential diagnoses.
- Discuss, OHSS, classified.
- Justify, examination, investigations.

Essay plan

A

- Other gynaecological causes e.g. ectopic.
- Other surgical causes e.g. appendicitis.

B

- Mild OHSS.
- Moderate OHSS.
- Severe OHSS.
- Critical OHSS.

C

- Examination – general, cardiovascular, pelvic.
- Investigation – bloods (FBC, U&Es, LFT), USS, CXR.

Suggested answer

A

It is important to consider other gynaecological and surgical causes of similar symptoms. An ectopic pregnancy or acute pelvic inflammatory disease should be excluded (1). Ovarian accidents such as torsion or rupture of an ovarian cyst may also present with similar symptoms (1). Surgical causes such as appendicitis and other bowel-related problems should also be considered (1).

B

Ovarian hyperstimulation syndrome (OHSS) is generally classified according to the severity of symptoms into mild, moderate, severe and critical (1). In mild OHSS the symptoms are of mild abdominal pain and abdominal bloating, and on ultrasound scan (USS) the ovarian size is usually under 8 cm (1). In moderate OHSS the patient complains of moderate abdominal pain and nausea with or without vomiting (1). USS shows evidence of ascites and the ovarian size is between 8 cm and 12 cm (1). Severe OHSS occurs when the patient presents with clinical ascites (occasional hydrothorax) and oliguria and the ovarian size is greater than 12 cm on USS (1). This is associated with a haematocrit of over 45% and hypoproteinaemia (1). OHSS is considered critical when the patient has tense ascites or large hydrothorax with oligo- or anuria and thromboembolism (1). This is associated with a haematocrit of greater than 55% and a white cell count of greater than 25,000 per ml (1). Acute respiratory distress syndrome can occur in this situation (1).

C

In suspected OHSS the examination must identify or exclude dehydration, enlarged ovaries, ascites and any signs of thromboembolism (1). A full cardiovascular and respiratory examination is needed to check for pericardial effusion or hydrothorax (1). The blood pressure, pulse rate and respiratory rate must be recorded (1). Any degree of dehydration needs to be noted and abdominal girth and weight measured (1). Investigations include a full blood count for haemoglobin concentration, haematocrit and white cell count, which may indicate dehydration and a predisposition to thromboembolism (1). Urea, electrolytes and liver function tests are performed to check for severity of dehydration affecting renal and liver function (1). A pelvic ultrasound scan checks for ovarian size and ascites (1). A chest radiograph, electrocardiogram (ECG) and echocardiogram need to be arranged if a hydrothorax or pericardial effusion is suspected (1).

Further reading

Royal College of Obstetricians and Gynaecologists. *The Management of Ovarian Hyperstimulation Syndrome.* Green-Top Guideline No. 5. London: RCOG, September 2006.

Shetty A. Disorders of ovulation. In: Bhattacharya S, Hamilton M, eds. *Management of Infertility for the MRCOG and Beyond.* London: RCOG Press, 2006: 43–64.

1.2.25 Chronic pelvic pain

A Define chronic pelvic pain. (2 marks)
B How would you manage a patient with chronic pelvic pain? (18 marks)

Key words in the question

- Define, chronic pelvic pain.
- Manage, chronic pelvic pain.

Essay plan

A

- Definition.

B

- Time to assess patient.
- History and pelvic examination, screen for infection.
- Abnormal pelvic exam, ultrasound $+/-$ laparoscopy.
- Normal pelvic exam, treat cause, symptoms.
- Laparoscopy $=$ 2nd line, diagnose endometriosis and adhesions.
- Essential to discuss with patient possibility of negative laparoscopy prior to surgery.

Suggested answer

A

Chronic pelvic pain (CPP) is defined as constant or intermittent pain in the lower abdomen or pelvis which has been present for at least six months, not associated with pregnancy and not occurring exclusively with menstruation or intercourse. It is a symptom and not a diagnosis (2).

B

It is important to let the patient tell her story, so sufficient time should be set aside for assessment. There is evidence that favourable patient rating at initial consultation results in a higher complete recovery rate at follow-up (1). The history should include questions about the pattern of the pain and any association with bladder, bowel and psychological symptoms and the effect of movement and posture on the pain (1). Symptoms suggestive of serious disease, e.g. rectal or postcoital bleeding, should be excluded (1). A history of past or present sexual assault or abuse is important, as CPP is commoner in these patients (1). Pelvic examination is important, to exclude pelvic or adnexal masses (1). It also offers the opportunity to screen for infection, e.g. gonorrhoea and chlamydia, if pelvic inflammatory disease (PID) is suspected. If PID is present, it is best treated by referring the woman to the genitourinary clinic so that appropriate microbiological advice and contact tracing can be arranged (1).

If pelvic examination is abnormal, an urgent ultrasound scan with or without diagnostic laparoscopy is arranged (1). If the clinical findings are normal, the multifactorial nature of CPP should be discussed and explored with the patient. It is helpful to develop a good relationship with her to plan appropriate management (1).

If the history suggests there is a significant non-gynaecological component to the pain, referral to the appropriate specialist, e.g. urologist, gastroenterologist or physiotherapist, should be considered (1).

If symptoms suggest irritable bowel syndrome (IBS), this is treated with high-fibre diet and an antispasmodic, such as mebeverine. If pain is inadequately controlled, the patient may be referred to the pain management team or specialist pelvic pain clinic (1).

If urogenital or other bowel symptoms predominate, the woman should be given analgesia and referred to a urologist or gastroenterologist (1).

If she has a marked psychological component to her pain, she can be commenced on analgesics and referred to a psychologist or psychiatrist (1).

If her pain varies with movement and nerve entrapment is suspected, a local anaesthetic injection may help (1). If the pain is predominantly musculoskeletal, physiotherapy is likely to be beneficial (1).

Should the patient have marked cyclical pain with dysmenorrhoea, a trial of combined oral contraception or gonadotrophin-releasing hormone (GnRH) analogue with analgesia for three to six months should help (1).

Laparoscopy is best reserved as a second-line investigation for CPP, provided the woman has a normal pelvic examination and/or ultrasound scan. Laparoscopy is useful for diagnosing endometriosis and adhesions (1). One-third to one-half of diagnostic laparoscopies are negative and pathology identified may not always be the cause of the patient's pain. It is very important to discuss the possibility of a negative laparoscopy with the woman prior to surgery (1). Laparoscopy is probably best reserved for those women who want to know whether they have endometriosis or adhesions that potentially could affect fertility or when the index of suspicion of finding endometriosis or adhesions is high (1).

Further reading

Royal College of Obstetricians and Gynaecologists. *The Initial Management of Chronic Pelvic Pain.* Green-Top Guideline No. 41. London: RCOG, April 2005.

SECTION 2
PRACTICE PAPERS

Paper 1

2.1.1.1

You have been called to the labour ward to review a primigravid woman who has just been delivered and sustained an anal sphincter injury.

A Discuss the classification of obstetric perineal injuries. (5 marks)

B Outline the principles of repair. (10 marks)

C What would be your advice regarding subsequent pregnancies? (5 marks)

2.1.1.2

A A 31-year-old patient books for antenatal care at 12 weeks. Her new partner has a child with cystic fibrosis from a previous relationship. The patient has no family history of cystic fibrosis. How would you counsel this patient? (10 marks)

B A 21-year-old patient with cystic fibrosis attends the antenatal clinic at 10 weeks' gestation. Discuss your plan of management for her antenatal care and delivery. (10 marks)

2.1.1.3

A Define domestic violence. (2 marks)

B What is the incidence of domestic violence in pregnancy and when is the risk of moderate to severe violence highest? (2 marks)

C What are the fetal risks of domestic violence? (3 marks)

D What would make you suspect domestic violence? (6 marks)

E Why are women thought to stay in a violent relationship? (7 marks)

2.1.1.4

A 40-year-old woman with a body mass index (BMI) of 41 kg/m^2 books for antenatal care at 12 weeks' gestation. She informs you she has been overweight for many years.

A Outline possible antenatal complications related to her BMI. (10 marks)

B During labour and delivery, what problems are more likely to be encountered than in a patient with a BMI of 25 kg/m^2? (10 marks)

Paper 2

2.1.2.1

A 35-year-old woman presents with symptoms of urgency, frequency, nocturia and urge incontinence. She does not complain of stress incontinence.

A Justify your initial investigations and non-surgical management. Do not discuss drug treatment. (7 marks)

B What advice would you give her with regard to lifestyle interventions? (7 marks)

C Identify three pharmacological agents used to treat the overactive bladder. Choose one medication and outline what precautions you would take before prescribing it and its common side effects. (6 marks)

2.1.2.2

You are the registrar assigned to the day surgical list. On the list is Mrs Smith, a 34-year-old woman, for laparoscopic clip sterilization.

A What information do you need to obtain from Mrs Smith prior to obtaining consent, and why? (5 marks)

B What advice would you give Mrs Smith regarding contraception? (6 marks)

C What are the serious risks involved in this type of surgery? (6 marks)

D Outline three types of failure of sterilization. (3 marks)

2.1.2.3

A How may a patient present as an emergency with ovarian cancer and why? (6 marks)

B If a patient presents with suspected ovarian cancer, what investigations would you arrange and why? (10 marks)

C What is the aim of primary surgery in ovarian cancer and what are the usual procedures performed? (4 marks)

2.1.2.4

A 16-year-old girl presents to the gynaecology outpatient clinic with a history of never having had a period.

A Define amenorrhoea. (2 marks)

B Outline the likely causes of the amenorrhoea in this case. (5 marks)

C What are the secondary sexual characteristics in a woman? (5 marks)

D Discuss cryptomenorrhoea. What is the likely cause, how does it present and how would you treat it? (8 marks)

Paper 1

2   **2.1.1.1**

You have been called to the labour ward to review a primigravid woman who has just been delivered and sustained an anal sphincter injury.

A   Discuss the classification of obstetric perineal injuries. (5 marks) *not just 4°p Tear*
B   Outline the principles of repair. (10 marks)
C   What would be your advice regarding subsequent pregnancies? (5 marks)

Key words in the question

- Primigravid, anal sphincter injury.
- Classification.
- Principles of repair.
- Advice.

Essay plan

A

- Discuss types of obstetric perineal injuries 1st, 2nd, 3rd (a, b, c) and 4th degree.

B

- Establish diagnosis.
- Outline where and who should undertake repair.
- Discuss surgical technique and choice of suture materials.
- Discuss aftercare.

C

- Recognize patient anxiety and concerns.
- Discuss prognosis.
- Give advice on management of delivery in future pregnancies.

Suggested answer

A

Obstetric anal sphincter tears have been classified by Sultan and adopted by the RCOG.
   First-degree tears involve injury to the perineal skin only (1).
   Second-degree tears involve perineal skin and muscles (1).
   Third-degree tears involve the anal sphincter complex and can be subdivided into: 3a, where less than 50% of the external anal sphincter (EAS) thickness is torn; 3b, where more than 50% of the EAS is torn; and 3c, where both the EAS and the internal anal sphincter (IAS) are torn (2).

Fourth-degree tears involve injury to the anal sphincter complex and the anal epithelium (1).

B

The patient should be examined by an experienced practitioner trained in the recognition and management of perineal tears, and Sultan's classification should be used (1).

Once the diagnosis has been made, the patient should be transferred to theatre for repair. The repair is performed under aseptic conditions with appropriate assistance, instruments and a good light source to provide optimal visualization. The use of regional or general anaesthesia allows the sphincter to relax, permitting the retrieval of the retracted torn muscle. It also allows the ends to be brought together without tension (2).

The two methods of repair of EAS are the end-to-end and the overlap technique. There is no evidence to recommend one technique over the other. Where the internal sphincter is damaged and can be recognized, it should be repaired separately with interrupted sutures. For repair of both the EAS and the IAS, either monofilament sutures such as polydiaxanone sutures (PDS) or modern braided sutures such as polyglactin (Vicryl) can be used with equivalent outcome. Fine sutures such as 3–0 PDS and 2–0 Vicryl may cause less irritation and discomfort. Knots should be buried beneath superficial muscles to prevent knot migration, although women should be warned that this can still occur (3).

Postoperatively women should be given broad-spectrum antibiotics and laxatives to reduce the incidence of infection and wound dehiscence (1).

Physiotherapy with pelvic floor exercises should be offered to all women for 6–12 weeks after repair (1).

All women who have sustained a third- or fourth-degree tear should be reviewed by a consultant obstetrician and gynaecologist between 6 and 12 weeks postpartum (1).

If the patient has incontinence or pain, referral to a specialist clinic is recommended for further investigations such as endoanal ultrasound and anal manometry (1).

C

Given the nature of the injury the woman's anxiety should be acknowledged (1).

The prognosis following EAS repair is good, with 60–80% of patients being asymptomatic at 12 months. Where women are symptomatic the symptoms tend to be of flatal incontinence or fecal urgency (2).

Women should be counselled about the risk of developing anal incontinence or worsening symptoms with subsequent vaginal delivery. There is no evidence to support the role of prophylactic episiotomy. If a woman is symptomatic or has abnormal endoanal ultrasound or anal manometry, she should be given the option of delivery by elective caesarean section (2).

Further reading

Royal College of Obstetricians and Gynaecologists. *The Management of Third and Fourth Degree Perineal Tears*. Green-Top Guideline No. 29. London. RCOG, March 2007.

2.1.1.2

A A 31-year-old patient books for antenatal care at 12 weeks. Her new partner has a child with cystic fibrosis from a previous relationship. The patient has no family history of cystic fibrosis. How would you counsel this patient? (10 marks)

B A 21-year-old patient with cystic fibrosis attends the antenatal clinic at 10 weeks' gestation. Discuss your plan of management for her antenatal care and delivery. (10 marks)

Key words in the question

- Books, 12 weeks, partner, child with cystic fibrosis, previous relationship, counsel.
- Cystic fibrosis, 10 weeks' gestation, plan of management, antenatal care, delivery.

Essay plan

A
- CF = autosomal recessive, partner = carrier. General population risk 1/22.
- Risk to this pregnancy 1/88. Pedigree and urgent referral to medical geneticist.
- Screen patient for CF. If screen negative then risk to pregnancy 1/880. Screen positive then risk 1/4 – offer prenatal diagnosis.

B
- Ascertain severity, liaise with physician. Assess respiratory function.
- Fetus at least a carrier – offer screening to partner. If positive, offer prenatal diagnosis.
- Chest problems – urgent medical review. Penicillin and bronchodilators safe. Risk of DM.
- Serial USS – IUGR risk. Preterm delivery common. Aim for vaginal delivery, epidural preferred. Prophylactic instrumental delivery.

Suggested answer

A

Since cystic fibrosis (CF) is an autosomal recessive condition, the patient's partner must be a carrier (1). This woman has no family history of CF, so she has the general population risk of 1 in 22 of being a carrier for CF (1). The risk of this pregnancy being affected by CF is 1 in 88 (1) [22 (her chance of being a carrier) × 1 (her partner is a carrier) × 4 (chance of parents who are both carriers passing on the relevant gene)]. I would inform the woman of the above information, drawing a pedigree/family tree to explain more easily the autosomal recessive nature of CF. I would also arrange urgent referral to a medical geneticist for more detailed counselling (2).

The risk of this patient having a baby with CF can be further assessed by screening the woman for CF carrier status. This involves a mouthwash sample, which is sent for DNA analysis. This tests for the commonest types of CF mutations, e.g. delF508, and detects 90% of mutations (2). Should the patient accept screening, and the result be negative, the risk of her being a carrier falls to 1 in 220 [1 in 22 × 1 in 10 − 10% of carriers are not detected by screening due to rare mutations], and the risk of her carrying a baby with CF falls to 1 in 880 (1) [1 in 220 × 1 (partner carrier) × 4 (1 in 4 chance of two carriers having a child with CF in autosomal recessive condition)]. Should she be screen positive, I would offer her prenatal diagnosis by fetal DNA analysis (either chorionic villous sampling or amniocentesis) (1). I would emphasize to the couple that should she undergo prenatal diagnosis she would not be put under pressure to have a termination of pregnancy if the fetus has CF. I would, however, inform them that termination of pregnancy is an option should they so desire (1).

B

I would take a comprehensive history from the patient to ascertain the severity of her CF, particularly her respiratory and nutritional status. Almost certainly she will be well known to a respiratory physician and I would liaise with him/her, as a multidisciplinary approach is essential (1). I would check that the patient is aware that pregnancy may be very challenging for her, especially if she has moderate or severe respiratory symptoms (1). Her respiratory function should be assessed, as this is a very useful predictor of outcome. If her forced expiratory volume (FEV_1) is >80%, a normal outcome is likely. If the FEV_1 is <50%, there is a high risk of maternal mortality, and it would be prudent to discuss termination of pregnancy with the patient (1). This baby will be at least a carrier for CF. Her partner should be offered screening for CF mutations if not already done. If her partner is screen positive, the woman may opt to have prenatal diagnosis with chorionic villous sampling or amniocentesis. Should her baby have CF, the option of termination of pregnancy may be considered (1).

If or when she develops chest problems, the respiratory physician should urgently review the woman. She will likely require regular chest physiotherapy. Should antibiotics be required, penicillin and cephalosporins are safe in pregnancy (1). Bronchodilators can also be used safely. Early referral into hospital should be arranged if problems occur (1). The woman may have malnutrition due to pancreatic insufficiency. She may have or develop diabetes mellitus; if so, a diabetologist should be involved in her care (1). She should have serial ultrasound scans to monitor fetal growth, as intrauterine growth retardation (IUGR) is common. Preterm delivery may be required due to IUGR (1).

Normal vaginal delivery is the aim. Epidural is the analgesia of choice. It is best to avoid general anaesthesia due to its respiratory effects (1). An instrumental delivery is recommended to shorten the second stage and reduce maternal compromise (1).

Further reading

Connor MJ. *Medical Genetics for the MRCOG and Beyond*. London: RCOG Press, 2005.
Crocker SG. MRCOG Part 2 model essay answer. *Current Obstetrics and Gynaecology* 2006; **16**: 64.

2.1.1.3

A Define domestic violence. (2 marks)

B What is the incidence of domestic violence in pregnancy and when is the risk of moderate to severe violence highest? (2 marks)

C What are the fetal risks of domestic violence? (3 marks)

D What would make you suspect domestic violence? (6 marks)

E Why are women thought to stay in a violent relationship? (7 marks)

Key words in the question

- Define domestic violence.
- Incidence, risk, moderate to severe, highest.
- Fetal risks.
- Suspect domestic violence.
- Why, women, stay, violent relationship.

Essay plan

A
- Intentional abuse, intimate relationship.
- Physical, sexual, psychological.

B
- 20%.
- Postpartum.

C
- Miscarriage, death, abruption, injury, prematurity, IUGR.

D
- Injuries, poor attenders, recurrent presentations, domineering partner.

E
- Fear, financial, family, faith, father, forgiveness, fatigue.

Suggested answer

A

Domestic violence is defined as the intentional abuse inflicted on one partner by another while in an intimate relationship (1). The abuse may be physical, sexual or psychological (1).

B

The incidence of domestic violence in pregnancy has been estimated as up to 20% (1). The risk of moderate to severe violence is at its highest in the postpartum period (1).

C

The risks to the fetus include miscarriage, intrauterine fetal death, placental abruption, fetal injury, preterm delivery and low birthweight (3).

D

A number of factors raise the index of suspicion of domestic violence, the leading one being injuries to the woman herself. Women suffering domestic violence tend to trivialize these injuries (1). [The injuries are classically to the pregnant abdomen, genitals and breasts.] The mechanism of injury often does not fit the type of injury noticed (1). The injuries may present late and there may be injuries of different ages (1). Women may book late and then be poor attenders at the antenatal clinic (1). Some women repeatedly present with seemingly trivial symptoms and are then reluctant to be discharged home (1). The partner is usually present and will often speak for the woman, who may be reluctant to speak herself (1).   *domineering partner*

E

The reasons for a woman remaining in a violent relationship are often multiple. They include fear, where the woman is frightened that she will be exposed to worse violence or even be killed if she leaves her partner (1). Financial reasons may be present, particularly if the partner has control of the woman's resources (1). There may be family (1) and faith (1) pressures to remain with the partner, and she may want to have a father figure for her children (1). Often the abuser will be sorry after the event of violence, promising that it will never happen again, and the woman forgives the partner (1). The woman may feel unable to do anything about the abuse due to low self-esteem and the stress of her situation ['fatigue'] (1).

Further reading

Baccus L, Bewley S, Mezey G. Domestic violence and pregnancy. *The Obstetrician and Gynaecologist* 2001; 3: 56–9.
Masson G. Domestic violence. In: Grady K, Howell C, Cox C, eds. *Managing Obstetric Emergencies and Trauma. The MOET Course Manual* (2nd edition). London: RCOG, 2007: 315–20.

2.1.1.4

A 40-year-old woman with a body mass index (BMI) of 41 kg/m^2 books for antenatal care at 12 weeks' gestation. She informs you she has been overweight for many years.

A   Outline possible antenatal complications related to her BMI. (10 marks)

B   During labour and delivery, what problems are more likely to be encountered than in a patient with a BMI of 25 kg/m^2? (10 marks)

Key words in the question

- 40-year-old, BMI, 41 kg/m^2, 12 weeks' gestation, overweight, many years.
- Antenatal complications.
- Labour and delivery, problems, more likely.

Essay plan

A

- Malformations, USS dating and anomaly more difficult, prenatal diagnosis more difficult.
- Abdominal palpation – may miss large or small baby.
- Gestational DM and PET more common.
- Fetal macrosomia and prolonged pregnancy more likely.

B

- FSE if external FM difficult.
- Increased risk instrumental and CS delivery with their obesity risks.
- Anaesthetic risks increased.

Suggested answer

A

This woman is at an increased risk of having a major fetal malformation (1). Due to her obesity abdominal ultrasound examination is more difficult to perform and interpret. Dating (1) and anomaly scanning may therefore be less accurate (1). Should she require prenatal diagnosis (possible since she is aged 40 years), this is technically more difficult and there is a threefold increase in miscarriage risks in the obese patient (1). In the third trimester, this patient's obesity will make abdominal palpation to determine fetal lie and presentation and symphyseal–fundal height less useful (1). This increases the risk of failing to detect a small or large baby (1).

This woman is more likely to develop gestational diabetes (1) and pre-eclampsia (1) than her counterpart with a normal BMI. She also is at a higher risk of having fetal macrosomia (1) and a prolonged pregnancy necessitating induction of labour (1).

B

During labour, it may be difficult to perform external fetal heart rate monitoring due to adipose tissue. Utilizing a fetal scalp electrode once the membranes are ruptured may help overcome this problem (1). She is more likely to require an instrumental delivery (1) or caesarean section (1). If she has a vaginal delivery, she is at increased risk of a third-degree tear compared with a patient with a normal BMI (1). This woman's baby is at increased risk of shoulder dystocia and brachial plexus injury, as obesity is associated with fetal macrosomia (2). Should she have any vaginal or cervical tears, these are often more difficult to identify and suture due to limited access and excessive vaginal adipose tissue (1). She is three times more likely to have a caesarean section for delay in the first stage of labour, and the operation itself will likely take significantly longer than if the woman had a normal BMI (1). Should she wish to have an epidural during labour, the siting of this or a spinal anaesthetic would be more difficult due to the increased distance from skin to the intervertebral space. Failure to achieve a suitable anaesthetic block is therefore more likely (1). If she requires a general anaesthetic, she has a higher risk of failed intubation (1).

Further reading

Fraser RB. Obesity complicating pregnancy. *Current Obstetrics and Gynaecology* 2006; **16**: 295–8.

Irvine L, Shaw R. The impact of obesity on obstetric outcomes. *Current Obstetrics and Gynaecology* 2006; **16**: 242–6.

Paper 2

2.1.2.1

A 35-year-old woman presents with symptoms of urgency, frequency, nocturia and urge incontinence. She does not complain of stress incontinence.

A Justify your initial investigations and non-surgical management. Do not discuss drug treatment. (7 marks)

B What advice would you give her with regard to lifestyle interventions? (7 marks)

C Identify three pharmacological agents used to treat the overactive bladder. Choose one medication and outline what precautions you would take before prescribing it and its common side effects. (6 marks)

Key words in the question

- 35-year-old, urgency, urge incontinence, not complain of stress incontinence.
- Justify, initial investigations, non-surgical management. Do not discuss drug treatment.
- Advice, lifestyle interventions.
- Three pharmacological agents, precautions, before prescribing, side effects.

Essay plan

A
- Urinalysis, MSU for C&S, antibiotics if positive culture.
- Urinary diary.
- Conservative treatment – bladder training.
- Urodynamics not recommended initially.

B
- Lose weight if BMI $>30 \text{ kg/m}^2$.
- Avoid caffeine, stop smoking, reduce alcohol.
- Fluid intake 1.5–2 litres/day.
- Timed voiding, review medications.
- Regular review with continence nurse specialist.

C
- Oxybutynin, tolterodine, solifenacin.
- Avoid myasthenia gravis, bladder outflow obstruction, severe ulcerative colitis.
- Caution in elderly, autonomic neuropathy and angle-closure glaucoma.
- Side effects – dry mouth, dry eyes, blurred vision, constipation, drowsiness, dizziness and difficulty in micturition.

Suggested answer

A

Appropriate initial investigations include a urine dipstick to detect blood, glucose, protein, leucocytes and nitrites. If the dipstick is positive for leucocytes and nitrites, a mid-stream specimen of urine (MSU) should be sent for culture and sensitivity analysis (1). Antibiotics should be prescribed only if infection is present (1).

The woman should be asked to keep a frequency/volume chart (urinary diary) for three days. A three-day period allows variation in day-to-day activities to be documented while securing reasonable compliance (1). This is a reliable method of quantifying urinary frequency, incontinence episodes, volumes ingested and voided. It can detect cases of excessive drinking, which may account for her symptoms of urgency, frequency and nocturia (1).

This patient should be commenced on conservative treatment (1). Bladder training for a minimum of six weeks should be offered as first-line treatment [see NICE Guideline No. 40]. Bladder training is effective treatment and has fewer adverse effects and lower relapse rates than antimuscarinic drugs (1).

Urodynamic investigation is not recommended before starting conservative treatment. Urodynamics is best reserved for cases before surgery if there is clinical suspicion of detrusor overactivity, symptoms suggestive of voiding dysfunction or previous failed surgery (1).

B

I would advise her to lose weight if her BMI is above $30 \, kg/m^2$ and offer referral to a dietician (1). She should avoid caffeine, which is present in tea and coffee. She should be advised to switch to decaffeinated products (1). Reduction in alcohol intake (if significant) and stopping smoking (as chronic coughing exacerbates incontinence) may also help (1). She should ensure her fluid intake is between 1.5 and 2 litres per day on average (1). Timed voiding can also help in retraining the bladder (1). Her current medications, e.g. diuretics, should be reviewed and if possible stopped or changed if they exacerbate her symptoms (1). Since lifestyle changes and bladder retraining are associated with a high relapse rate, this woman should maintain regular contact with the continence nurse specialist, who will be able to encourage and reinforce these changes (1).

C

Three pharmacological agents used to treat the overactive bladder are oxybutynin, tolterodine and solifenacin (1). [Other possibilities include trospium chloride, darifenacin, propantheline and propiverine hydrochloride.]

Immediate-release oxybutynin is recommended as first-line treatment by the National Institute for Health and Clinical Excellence. It should be avoided in patients with myasthenia gravis, significant bladder outflow obstruction or urinary retention, severe ulcerative colitis or gastrointestinal obstruction (2). Caution is advisable in the elderly, in patients with autonomic neuropathy and those susceptible to angle-closure glaucoma (1).

Common side effects include dry mouth, dry eyes, blurred vision, constipation, drowsiness, dizziness and difficulty in micturition (2).

Further reading

Drugs for urinary frequency, enuresis, and incontinence, section 7.4.2. *British National Formulary* (BNF), No. 52, March 2008: 440–3.

Foon R, Toozs-Hobson P. Detrusor overactivity. *Obstetrics, Gynaecology and Reproductive Medicine* 2007; **17**: 255–60.

National Institute for Health and Clinical Excellence. *The Management of Urinary Incontinence in Women*. NICE Clinical Guideline No. 40. London: NICE, October 2006.

2.1.2.2

You are the registrar assigned to the day surgical list. On the list is Mrs Smith, a 34-year-old woman, for laparoscopic clip sterilization.

A What information do you need to obtain from Mrs Smith prior to obtaining consent, and why? (5 marks)

B What advice would you give Mrs Smith regarding contraception? (6 marks)

C What are the serious risks involved in this type of surgery? (6 marks)

D Outline three types of failure of sterilization. (3 marks)

Key words in the question

- Information, prior to, consent.
- Advice, contraception.
- Serious risks.
- Three types, failure, sterilization.

Essay plan

A
- History, date of LMP, current contraception, pregnancy test.

B
- Continue contraception, discuss type and when to stop.

C
- Risks related to laparoscopy and risks related to sterilization.

D
- Pre-existing pregnancy, early operative technical failure or late failure.

Suggested answer

A

A thorough history should be obtained on the day of surgery, to include the date of the last menstrual period (LMP), the type of contraception currently being used by Mrs Smith, and her surgical and sexual history (3).

This will allow me to decide whether Mrs Smith is at risk of either being or getting pregnant. If her period is late, it is essential to perform a pregnancy test. If she is in the luteal phase of her cycle having had unprotected intercourse, then she needs to be counselled regarding the risk of becoming pregnant and her operation may need to be postponed (2).

B

It is important to inform Mrs Smith of the need to continue with an effective method of contraception in the menstrual cycle in which the operation takes place. This is to ensure that pregnancy does not occur around the time of the sterilization (1).

If she uses a barrier method of contraception, then she should continue to use this until her next period after the sterilization (1).

Should Mrs Smith be using a hormonal method of contraception, then she should be told to carry on taking the pills until the end of the current packet or, in the case of the progesterone-only pill, the end of the next packet or her next period, whichever is sooner (2).

If Mrs Smith's method of contraception is an intrauterine device, then this should be removed at her next period. If she uses the levonorgestrel-releasing system, then it should be removed at least seven days after the sterilization has been performed (2).

C

The serious risks involved in laparoscopic clip sterilization are failure of sterilization (1/200), the risk of this failure resulting in an ectopic pregnancy, the failure to gain access to the abdomen, perforation of the uterus, injuries to viscera such as bowel and blood vessels (3/1000 procedures), and death (1/12,000) (6).

D

There are three recognized types of failure of sterilization. The first is a pre-existing pregnancy, either in a previous cycle or a luteal-phase pregnancy in the current one (1).

The second is early technical and operative failure, where failure occurs as a result of poor technique, including only partial application of the clip or ring, or its application to the wrong structure (1).

The last is late failure, which can occur even after the correct technique is performed, when recannulization occurs (1).

Further reading

Roberts N, Argent V. Avoiding pregnancy at the time of sterilisation. *The Obstetrician and Gynaecologist* 2004; **6**: 159–62.

Royal College of Obstetricians and Gynaecologists. *Laparoscopic Tubal Occlusion*. Consent Advice No. 3. London: RCOG, October 2004.

2.1.2.3

A How may a patient present as an emergency with ovarian cancer and why? (6 marks)

B If a patient presents with suspected ovarian cancer, what investigations would you arrange and why? (10 marks)

C What is the aim of primary surgery in ovarian cancer and what are the usual procedures performed? (4 marks)

Key words in the question

- Present, emergency, ovarian cancer, why.
- Suspected ovarian cancer, investigations, why.
- Aim, primary surgery, ovarian cancer, what, usual procedures.

Essay plan

A
- Pain, distension, raised intra-abdominal pressure, pressure effects.

B
- Bloods – FBC, U&E, LFT, CA125.
- Imaging – CXR. USS pelvis, CT.

C
- Confirm diagnosis, stage, remove.
- TAH, BSO, omentectomy, LN sampling and washings.

Suggested answer

A

Patients with ovarian cancer may present as an emergency with a variety of symptoms. They can present with abdominal pain due to torsion or ischaemia of the cancer (1). Patients may complain of rapid abdominal distension, which may be due to the tumour growth or to associated ascites (1). Distension is also associated with acute and subacute bowel obstruction, which may be due to pressure of the tumour or infiltration of the bowel itself (1). Increasing intra-abdominal pressure may cause respiratory compromise, with breathlessness and prolapse (2). The ureters can be involved either by infiltration or via direct pressure, and this may present as renal failure (1).

B

In the case of suspected ovarian cancer, I would arrange blood tests, including full blood count (FBC), urea and electrolytes (U&Es), liver function tests (LFTs) and tumour markers such as cancer antigen 125 (CA125) (1). The FBC is important, as this patient may be anaemic and require surgery (1). The U&Es assess renal function and the LFTs help exclude liver infiltration (2). CA125 is raised in the majority of patients with ovarian cancer, and while it has no prognostic value when measured at the time of diagnosis, it is used to monitor response to chemotherapy. If it normalizes and then subsequently begins to rise again, this is associated with tumour recurrence (2).

Imaging which is useful includes a chest radiograph, pelvic and abdominal ultrasound scan (USS) and computerized tomography (CT) (1). The chest radiograph may reveal a pleural effusion (1). The USS is a first-line investigation to confirm the clinical findings of an adnexal mass and its nature (solid or cystic) (1). A CT scan may help with planning the surgical resection, by delineating the tumour (1).

C

The aim of primary surgery in ovarian cancer is to confirm the diagnosis (1) and then to stage the disease using the FIGO classification (1) and to optimally debulk (or completely remove) the tumour (1). The usual operation undertaken is a total abdominal hysterectomy, bilateral salpingo-oophorect-omy and infra-colic omentectomy, with sampling of retroperitoneal lymph nodes and peritoneal washings (1).

Further reading

Luesley D, Achesen N, eds. *Gynaecological Oncology for the MRCOG and Beyond*. London: RCOG Press, 2004.

2.1.2.4

A 16-year-old girl presents to the gynaecology outpatient clinic with a history of never having had a period.

A Define amenorrhoea. (2 marks)

B Outline the likely causes of the amenorrhoea in this case. (5 marks)

C What are the secondary sexual characteristics in a woman? (5 marks)

D Discuss cryptomenorrhoea. What is the likely cause, how does it present and how would you treat it? (8 marks)

Key words in the question

- 16-year-old girl, never having had a period.
- Define amenorrhoea.
- Outline, causes, amenorrhoea.
- Secondary sexual characteristics.
- Discuss cryptomenorrhoea, likely cause, present, treat.

Essay plan

A
- Primary, secondary.

B
- Primary amenorrhoea.
- Primary – hormonal, delay, chronic disease, no ovarian function, hypothalamic – pituitary dysfunction.
- Anatomical – structural (absent), imperforate hymen.

C
- Breasts, hair, genital growth, hips, fat distribution.

D
- Definition, 1:4000, clinical features, treatment.

Suggested answer

A

Amenorrhoea can be categorized as primary and secondary. Primary amenorrhoea occurs when a girl has never experienced a menstrual period by the age of 16. Secondary amenorrhoea occurs with the absence of periods for more than six months (2).

B

As there has never been a period, this is a case of primary amenorrhoea. The causes are divided into those with the absence of secondary sexual characteristics and those where secondary sexual characteristics are present (1). The causes where there are no secondary sexual characteristics are usually hormonal and include constitutional delay, chronic systemic disease, the absence of ovarian function and hypothalamic pituitary dysfunction (2). In those cases where secondary sexual characteristics are present, the cause is usually anatomical and includes an absent uterus or endometrium, an absent vagina or an imperforate hymen (2).

C

The secondary sexual characteristics in a woman are breast development, growth of body hair, including pubic hair, and uterine and vaginal growth (3). There is a widening of the hips and a change in fat distribution, with deposition taking place around the buttocks, thighs and hips (2).

D

Cryptomenorrhoea is a condition which describes women who are menstruating, but in whom bleeding is concealed. (1). It occurs in 1 in 4000 girls (1). The likeliest cause is an imperforate hymen (1). It usually presents as acute abdominal pain and is often confused with appendicitis (1). Associated symptoms include urinary retention, due to pressure of collected blood, and a mass (1). Examination findings include a mass arising from the pelvis and a bulging blue membrane on parting the labia due to the haematocolpos (2). Treatment of an imperforate hymen is surgical via a cruciate incision to allow drainage of the menstrual blood (1).

Further reading

Garden AS, Topping J. *Paediatric and Adolescent Gynaecology for the MRCOG and Beyond*. London: RCOG Press, 2001.

Practice exam 2: Questions

Paper 1

2.2.1.1

A Define external cephalic version (ECV). (1 mark)

B What information would you give a woman at 36 weeks' gestation in the antenatal clinic with a breech presentation regarding ECV? (11 marks)

C What are the absolute contraindications to ECV (i.e. those associated with an increased risk of mortality or morbidity)? (4 marks)

D What are the relative contraindications to ECV (i.e. where ECV may be more difficult)? (4 marks)

2.2.1.2

A 28-year-old woman who is known to be HIV positive attends the antenatal booking clinic.

A She is worried about the risks to her baby. How can she be reassured? (4 marks)

B How should an HIV-positive woman be managed antenatally? (10 marks)

C What factors should to be taken into consideration in deciding on the mode of delivery? (6 marks)

2.2.1.3

A Discuss the risks associated with a prolonged but otherwise uncomplicated pregnancy. (3 marks)

B Discuss the recommendation from the National Institute for Health and Clinical Excellence (NICE) of offering induction of labour (IOL) in order to reduce these risks in prolonged pregnancy. (7 marks)

C If a woman declined IOL at the NICE-recommended gestation, how would you manage the rest of her pregnancy? Assume that the increased risks have been fully discussed with the patient. (3 marks)

D Discuss the modified Bishop's score. (7 marks)

2.2.1.4

A primigravid patient attends the antenatal assessment unit at 39 weeks' gestation with absent fetal movements for 24 hours. An ultrasound scan confirms an intrauterine death.

A How would you counsel the patient? (8 marks)

B What investigations would you arrange and why? (9 marks)

C Assuming no cause for the intrauterine death is found, how would you manage a subsequent pregnancy? (3 marks)

Paper 2

2.2.2.1

A What strategies could you use to reduce the long-term consequences of polycystic ovarian syndrome (PCOS) in an obese patient? (12 marks)

B When might surgery for a patient with PCOS be appropriate? (2 marks)

C Outline treatment options for hirsutism in an obese patient with PCOS. (6 marks)

2.2.2.2

A Discuss the risk factors for developing cervical cancer and preinvasive disease. (6 marks)

B What is cervical intraepithelial neoplasia (CIN) and what are the grading types? (4 marks)

C Which group is the target population for human papillomavirus (HPV) vaccination? (2 marks)

D What are the challenges for HPV vaccination and its acceptance? (6 marks)

E What is HPV vaccination's likely impact on cervical screening? (2 marks)

2.2.2.3

A 25-year-old Asian woman is admitted with a two-week history of severe nausea and vomiting at eight weeks' gestation.

A Justify your investigations. (7 marks)

B Hyperemesis is confirmed. Evaluate your management. (10 marks)

C What is Wernicke's encephalopathy and how may it be prevented? (3 marks)

2.2.2.4

A 54-year-old woman taking combined hormone replacement therapy (HRT) for three years to relieve vasomotor symptoms attends the gynaecological outpatient clinic, concerned about the risks of continuing on HRT.

A Describe the risks to this patient of her taking HRT. (7 marks)

B Outline the advantages of HRT. (7 marks)

C How would you ensure she makes an informed choice? (6 marks)

Practice exam 2: Answers

Paper 1

2.2.1.1

A Define external cephalic version (ECV). (1 mark)

B What information would you give a woman at 36 weeks' gestation in the antenatal clinic with a breech presentation regarding ECV? (11 marks)

C What are the absolute contraindications to ECV (i.e. those associated with an increased risk of mortality or morbidity)? (4 marks)

D What are the relative contraindications to ECV (i.e. where ECV may be more difficult)? (4 marks)

Key words in the question

A Define, ECV.

B Information, antenatal clinic, breech presentation, ECV.

C Absolute contraindications.

D Relative contraindications.

Essay plan

A

Define ECV.

B

Discuss how this patient will be counselled regarding timing, method, risks and success. What happens if it fails?

C

List absolute contraindications.

D

List relative contraindications.

Suggested answer

A

External cephalic version (ECV) is the manipulation of the fetus through the maternal abdomen to give a cephalic presentation (1).

B

I would introduce myself to the woman and discuss her options. I would outline what an ECV entails and inform her of the timing of the procedure (after 36 weeks' gestation) and that we offer this to increase the likelihood of her achieving a vaginal birth (2).

ECV is successful in approximately 50% of women. This chance may be increased if medication to relax the uterus is given, such as ritodrine or terbutaline (2).

ECV may be attempted twice but if the baby has not turned after the second attempt, other options for delivery (e.g. caesarean section) will be discussed with the patient (1).

ECV is generally safe but, as with any medical procedure, complications can occur. Premature labour does not seem to be associated with ECV. One in 200 babies need to be delivered after ECV due to a combination of bleeding from the placenta or changes in the baby's heartbeat. Monitoring of mother and baby will be carried out prior to, during and after the procedure (3).

ECV can be uncomfortable and the obstetrician will stop if you tell him or her it hurts. About 5% of patients report high pain scores (1).

If the patient experiences bleeding, abdominal pain, contractions or reduced movements following ECV, she should contact the hospital (2).

C

The absolute contraindications for ECV (i.e. factors likely to be associated with an increased risk of mortality or morbidity) include where caesarean section is required for another reason, antepartum haemorrhage in the last seven days, abnormal cardiotocogram, major uterine anomaly, ruptured membranes and multiple pregnancy (4).

D

The relative contraindications for ECV (where the procedure may be more complicated) include a fetus that is small for gestational age, abnormal Doppler ultrasound scans, proteinuric pre-eclampsia, oligohydramnios, major fetal anomalies, a scarred uterus and an unstable lie (4).

Further reading

Royal College of Obstetricians and Gynaecologists. *External Cephalic Version and Reducing the Incidence of Breech Presentation.* Green-Top Guideline No. 20a. London: RCOG, December 2006.

Royal College of Obstetricians and Gynaecologists. *Turning a Breech Baby in the Womb (External Cephalic Version): Information for You.* London: RCOG, February 2008.

2.2.1.2

A 28-year-old woman who is known to be HIV positive attends the antenatal booking clinic.

A She is worried about the risks to her baby. How can she be reassured? (4 marks)

B How should an HIV-positive woman be managed antenatally? (10 marks)

C What factors should to be taken into consideration in deciding on the mode of delivery? (6 marks)

Key words in the question

- HIV positive, worried about risks to her baby, reassured.
- How, HIV-positive, managed antenatally.
- Factors, mode of delivery.

Essay plan

A

- Antiretroviral treatment.
- Elective caesarean section delivery.
- Avoid breast-feeding.

B

- Multidisciplinary team management. Routine screening tests and anomaly scan.
- Antiretroviral treatment. If prenatal diagnosis, refer fetal medicine unit.
- Monitoring of plasma viral load and CD4 T-lymphocyte count.
- Prophylaxis for PCP.
- Single agent or combination therapy.
- Monitoring for maternal drug toxicity.
- Checking for other genital infections.

C

- Factors: on HAART and detectable viral load.
- Elective caesarean section or not at 38 weeks.
- If vaginal delivery, special considerations during labour.

Suggested answer

A

Since we know she is HIV positive, she should be reassured that measures can be put in place to decrease the risk of transmission of HIV to her unborn child. These measures include giving antiretroviral therapy during pregnancy and to the baby in the first six weeks of life (1). Delivery should be by elective caesarean section (1) and she should be advised to avoid breast-feeding (1). The implementation of these three interventions can reduce the vertical transmission rate of HIV from 30% to less than 2% (1).

B

This woman should be managed by a multidisciplinary team, including an obstetrician, HIV physician, midwife, paediatrician and possibly a psychiatric nurse (1).

She should be offered routine screening tests, including an anomaly scan at 20 weeks to detect any potential teratogenic effects of antiretroviral agents (1) If invasive screening tests such as amniocentesis or chorionic villus sampling are contemplated, the patient should be counselled and referred to a fetal medicine unit, as the risk of HIV transmission with these procedures is uncertain (1).

The plasma viral load and the CD4 T-lymphocyte count should be monitored regularly by the HIV physician, who will then advise regarding the choice and timing of antiretroviral therapy (1). Based on the CD4 count, prophylaxis against *Pneumocystis carinii* pneumonia (PCP) may be required (1). The choice of antiretroviral medication will be either a single agent with zidovudine (1) or combination therapy with highly active antiretroviral therapy (HAART) (1).

She should be monitored for drug toxicity by measuring full blood count, urea and electrolytes, liver function, lactate metabolism and blood glucose (1). Drug toxicity should be considered if the patient presents with liver dysfunction during the pregnancy (1).

Screening for genital tract infections should be performed and they must be treated appropriately if present. This is important because such infections may increase the local viral load and thus increase the risk of vertical transmission of HIV (1).

C

The main factors to consider are whether or not the patient is taking HAART or has a detectable plasma viral load (1). If the patient is not taking HAART or has a detectable plasma viral load, she should be offered elective caesarean section at 38 weeks because of the increased risk of vertical transmission (1). The morbidity from caesarean section in these patients is similar to that for HIV-negative patients except for a slightly increased risk of sepsis due to the mother's immunocompromised state (1).

However, if the patient is taking HAART or has an undetectable plasma viral load, the benefit of caesarean section is uncertain (1). These facts need to be discussed with the mother and her wishes considered. Should she opt for vaginal delivery, then prolonged labour, prolonged rupture of membranes, fetal blood sampling or use of fetal scalp electrodes should be avoided, and the cord should be clamped as soon as possible after birth and the baby washed immediately (2).

Further reading

Hawkins D, Blott M, Clayden P, *et al*. Guidelines for the management of HIV infection in pregnant women and the prevention of mother to child transmission of HIV. *HIV Medicine* 2005; 6 (suppl. 2): 107–48.

Royal College of Obstetricians and Gynaecologists. *Management of HIV in Pregnancy*. Green-Top Guideline No. 39. London: RCOG, April 2004.

2.2.1.3

2

A Discuss the risks associated with a prolonged but otherwise uncomplicated pregnancy. (3 marks)

B Discuss the recommendation from the National Institute for Health and Clinical Excellence (NICE) of offering induction of labour (IOL) in order to reduce these risks in prolonged pregnancy. (7 marks)

C If a woman declined IOL at the NICE-recommended gestation, how would you manage the rest of her pregnancy? Assume that the increased risks have been fully discussed with the patient. (3 marks)

D Discuss the modified Bishop's score. (7 marks)

Key words in the question

- Discuss, risks, prolonged, pregnancy.
- Discuss, recommendation, NICE, IOL, reduce, risks.

- Declined IOL, manage, pregnancy.
- Discuss, Bishop's score.

Essay plan

A

- Increased PN mortality and morbidity rate.

B

- IOL at 41 weeks.
- Reduced CS rate, no change instrumental delivery.
- Increased cost.

C

- Monitoring after 42 weeks – CTG and USS.

D

- Modified Bishop's score – 5 factors: cervical length, dilatation, station, consistency and position.

Suggested answer

A

The risks associated with a prolonged pregnancy are the increasing perinatal mortality and morbidity (1). The risk of stillbirth increases from 1 in 3000 continuing pregnancies at 37 weeks' gestation to 3 in 3000 at 42 weeks and 6 in 3000 at 43 weeks (1). There is a similar increase in neonatal mortality (1).

B

The National Institute for Health and Clinical Excellence (NICE) recommends offering induction of labour (IOL) in an otherwise uncomplicated pregnancy at 41 weeks' gestation (1). NICE analysed studies that looked at routine IOL versus expectant management. Routine IOL reduced the rate of caesarean section compared with conservative management after 41 weeks (1). There was no effect on the rates of instrumental delivery, use of epidural analgesia or fetal heart rate abnormalities (3). A reduction in meconium-stained liquor was also seen (1). A policy of routine IOL at 41 weeks would generate an increase in workload, which would need to be taken into consideration by the NHS (1).

C

I would recommend that this woman have increased monitoring after 42 weeks' gestation. This requires cardiotocography and ultrasound estimation of liquor volume twice weekly (3).

D

The modified Bishop's score is a pre-induction cervical assessment score (1). It consists of five components, which are the cervical length, cervical dilatation, the station of the presenting part relative to the ischial spines, the cervical consistency and the cervical position (5). These are scored from 0 to 3 and the maximum score attainable is 12. The higher the score, the more likely it is that IOL will be successful (1).

Further reading

National Institute for Clinical Excellence. *Induction of Labour*. Evidence-Based Clinical Guideline No. 9. London: NICE, June 2001.

2.2.1.4

A primigravid patient attends the antenatal assessment unit at 39 weeks' gestation with absent fetal movements for 24 hours. An ultrasound scan confirms an intrauterine death.

A How would you counsel the patient? (8 marks)

B What investigations would you arrange and why? (9 marks)

C Assuming no cause for the intrauterine death is found, how would you manage a subsequent pregnancy? (3 marks)

Key words in the question

- Primigravid, 39 weeks' gestation, absent fetal movements.
- Ultrasound, intrauterine death.
- How, counsel.
- Investigations, why.
- Manage, subsequent pregnancy.

Essay plan

A

- Quiet place, break news.
- Skill and empathy.
- Do not know why baby died – may know later.
- Explain IOL. Avoid CS if possible.
- Post-mortem.
- Home same day if all OK.

B

- Maternal bloods – FBC, blood group and antibody, infection screen TORCH, Kleihauer, U + Es, LFTs, HbA1c, APS, activated protein C resistance.
- Post-mortem, umbilical cord blood, placenta for histology.
- Thrombophilia screening.

C

- Offer 'reassurance' scans 28 and 34 weeks.
- IOL at 38 weeks.
- Reassure very unlikely SB will recur.

Suggested answer

A

I would ensure the patient was in a quiet room with family support if possible before breaking the news (1). I would inform the patient that tragically her baby's heart has stopped and she/he is no longer alive (1). Counselling in this situation requires skill and empathy, and I would endeavour to provide this with support from the attending midwife (1). Initially the mother and/or family usually express shock, confusion, disbelief and sometimes anger, and often ask why the baby has died. I would advise the woman that the cause of her baby dying is unknown at present, but we will try to find the cause in due course (1). At this stage I would offer to give the mother and her family some time together alone and return later to discuss delivery. I would explain the process of induction of labour and the advantages of a vaginal delivery (1) [it minimizes postnatal inpatient time and speeds up general recovery]. I would inform her that she can have an epidural or patient-controlled analgesia early in labour for pain relief and she will have access to a dedicated quiet room/bereavement suite with her partner and family (1). I would mention a post-mortem examination and briefly explain the advantages and disadvantages of her permitting her baby to have an autopsy. She does not need to make a decision regarding a post-mortem examination until after delivery (1). I would inform her that once delivered she will be able to go home quickly unless there is an unexpected complication (1).

B

Appropriate investigations include maternal blood tests for full blood count (for haemoglobin, and white-cell count for infection), infection screen (for cytomegalovirus, toxoplasmosis, parvovirus B19 and rubella and syphilis if not already taken in pregnancy), Kleihauer–Betke test for fetomaternal haemorrhage (regardless of blood group), HbA1c (to ascertain glucose control over previous six weeks), anticardiolipin antibodies and lupus anticoagulant (to test for antiphospholipid syndrome), bile salts (to exclude obstetric cholestasis) and activated protein C resistance. Maternal genital swabs should be taken if infection is suspected (4).

After delivery the baby should be sent for post-mortem examination if the patient gives consent. A post-mortem examination is the most important of all investigations offered, as new information becomes available in 40% of cases (2). Blood samples may be taken from the umbilical cord for investigations of infection and chromosomal analysis (1). The placenta should also be swabbed for infection and sent for histopathology (1).

A thrombophilia screen should be arranged two to three months post-partum if the intrauterine death was associated with fetal growth restriction or pre-eclampsia, if the stillbirth remains unexplained, or if tests for lupus anticoagulant or anticardiolipin antibodies were positive at delivery (1).

C

There are no evidence-based guidelines for the management of a subsequent pregnancy, so most management is based on professional experience. I would offer to see the woman and her partner regularly throughout pregnancy with 'reassurance' scans at 28 and 34 weeks' gestation (1). I would also offer induction of labour at 38 weeks (1). I would reassure the couple that it is very unlikely that she will experience a recurrence of stillbirth (1).

Further reading

Department of Health NSW Health Policy Directive. *Stillbirth – Management and Investigation*. Document number PD2007_025, April 2007. Accessed online at www.health.nsw.gov.au/policies/.

Luesley DM, Baker PN. Intrauterine fetal death. In: *Obstetrics and Gynaecology: An Evidence-Based Text for MRCOG*. London: Arnold, 2004: 317–24.

Paper 2

2.2.2.1

A What strategies could you use to reduce the long-term consequences of polycystic ovarian syndrome (PCOS) in an obese patient? (12 marks)

B When might surgery for a patient with PCOS be appropriate? (2 marks)

C Outline treatment options for hirsutism in an obese patient with PCOS. (6 marks)

Key words in the question

- Strategies, reduce, long-term consequences, PCOS, obese patient.
- Surgery, PCOS, appropriate.
- Treatment, hirsutism, obese.

Essay plan

A

- Reduce weight and increase exercise – drug therapy.
- Bariatric surgery.

B

- Ovarian drilling for anovulatory patient with normal BMI.
- Bariatric surgery for morbidly obese.

C

- Dianette, cosmetic measures, eflornithine cream.
- Others – metformin, spironolactone, reverse sequential regime.

Suggested answer

A

To reduce the long-term risks, this patient should be strongly encouraged to lose weight (diet) and to exercise more (30 minutes of sweat-inducing activity daily) (2). Loss of weight can improve fertility, as, often, spontaneous ovulation resumes (1). Weight reduction and exercise also reduce the risk of developing type II diabetes in later life by half (1).

Weight-reduction drugs, e.g. orlistat [a lipase inhibitor] or sibutramine [inhibits the reuptake of noradrenalin and serotonin], significantly reduce body weight and hyperandrogenism (1).

Metformin is unlicensed in polycystic ovarian syndrome (PCOS) and appears not to be superior to lifestyle interventions in improving cardio-metabolic risks and progression to type II diabetes mellitus (1).

Women with PCOS may have a higher cardiovascular risk than weight-matched women with normal ovaries (1). Such risks include obesity, hyper-androgenism, hyperlipidaemia and hyperinsulinaemia (1). Some of these factors are improved by lifestyle interventions (weight loss and exercise). Lipid-lowering drugs, e.g. statins, are not recommended unless prescribed by a specialist (1). Where present, hypertension should be treated (1).

Oligo- or amenorrhoea in women with PCOS may predispose to endo-metrial hyperplasia and carcinoma. A withdrawal bleed every three to four months, using cyclical progestogens, the oral contraceptive pill or Mirena, protects against this risk (1).

If the patient remains morbidly obese, then bariatric surgery may be considered (1).

B

Ovarian drilling should be performed only if a patient is anovulatory and has a normal body mass index or where laparoscopy is required for another reason (1).

Bariatric surgery, e.g. gastric banding, is reserved for the morbidly obese who fail to lose weight with diet, exercise and drug therapy (1).

C

Treatment options include Dianette (1) (combined oral contraceptive with cyproterone acetate), the topical facial cream eflornithine (1), and cosmetic procedures such as waxing, shaving, bleaching, laser and electrolysis (1). Often a combination of methods is required to achieve an acceptable cosmetic result (1). Unlicensed treatments include metformin, spironolactone and a reverse sequential regime of ethinyl oestradiol with 10–12 days per month of high-dose cyproterone acetate. Adequate contraceptive measures are essential with these medications (2).

Further reading

Royal College of Obstetricians and Gynaecologists. *Long-Term Consequences of Polycystic Ovary Syndrome.* Green-Top Guideline No. 33. London: RCOG, December 2007.

2.2.2.2

A Discuss the risk factors for developing cervical cancer and preinvasive disease. (6 marks)

B What is cervical intraepithelial neoplasia (CIN) and what are the grading types? (4 marks)

C Which group is the target population for human papillomavirus (HPV) vaccination? (2 marks)

D What are the challenges for HPV vaccination and its acceptance? (6 marks)

E What is HPV vaccination's likely impact on cervical screening? (2 marks)

Key words in the question

- Risk factors, cervical cancer, preinvasive disease.
- CIN, grading.
- Target population, HPV, vaccination.
- Challenges, HPV, vaccination.
- Impact, cervical screening.

Essay plan

A HPV 16 & 18, smoking, COCP.

B CIN 1, 2, 3.

C Adolescent girls.

D Public acceptability, public health campaigns, opposition groups, ?male vaccinations, ?booster doses.

E Some women may think don't need screening – still need screening.

Suggested answer

A

The risk factors associated with cervical cancer and preinvasive changes include human papillomavirus (HPV), particularly types 16 and 18. Early age at first intercourse and multiple sexual partners raise women's risk of contracting HPV, thereby increasing the risk of preinvasive and invasive disease (2).

There is an association with smoking, which may be related to a direct mutagenic effect upon cervical squamous cells, resulting in an impaired response to HPV infection (2).

Women who use the combined oral contraceptive pill are also at risk, and this is thought to be related to the metaplasia associated with the oestrogen. This risk is still present even when allowance is made for the increased chance of contracting HPV, given that these women are less likely than others to use barrier contraception (2).

B

Cervical intraepithelial neoplasia (CIN) describes the abnormal maturation and cytonuclear atypia which occur in the squamous epithelium of the cervix (1).

It has a three-tier grading system, CIN 1, 2 and 3. In CIN 1 the abnormality is confined to the basal third of the epithelium, in CIN 2 the abnormality occurs in the lower two-thirds, and in CIN 3 the abnormality occurs throughout (3).

C

The target population for HPV vaccination is adolescent girls before the start of sexual activity (2).

D

With the target population being adolescent girls before the start of sexual activity, the challenges include public acceptability (1).

Sensitive public health campaigns need to be in place to convince parents to vaccinate their daughters against a sexually transmitted infection (1).

There may be some groups who oppose vaccination on the grounds that it may promote promiscuity. Some are changing their position due to the chance of the husband introducing the HPV infection to their daughters after marriage (1).

The issue of whether boys should be vaccinated remains unresolved due to male disease being rare and there being no current work which demonstrates that vaccination can protect men (1).

There is no current indication as to whether booster HPV vaccination will be required. There are five-year data which have demonstrated that the immune response can last this long, but no longer-term data are yet available (2).

E

Concerns have been raised that the use of HPV vaccination could have an adverse effect on cervical screening if a woman believes she is now protected against cervical cancer (1). Cervical screening should be encouraged, as some women may not be fully protected and there will be women who have not been vaccinated (1).

Further reading

Luesely D, Acheson N, eds. *Gynaecological Oncology for the MRCOG and Beyond.* London: RCOG Press, 2004.

Royal College of Obstetricians and Gynaecologists. *Vaccination Against Cervical Cancer.* Scientific Advisory Committee Opinion Paper No. 9. London: RCOG, February 2007.

2.2.2.3

2 A 25-year-old Asian woman is admitted with a two-week history of severe nausea and vomiting at eight weeks' gestation.

A Justify your investigations. (7 marks)

B Hyperemesis is confirmed. Evaluate your management. (10 marks)

C What is Wernicke's encephalopathy and how may it be prevented? (3 marks)

Key words in the question

- Two-week history, severe nausea and vomiting, eight weeks' gestation.
- Justify, investigations.
- Hyperemesis, evaluate, management.
- Wernicke's encephalopathy, prevented.

Essay plan

A

- U&Es, FBC, LFTs, urinalysis, MSU, TFTs, USS.

B

- Fluid and electrolyte replacement – N saline, Hartmann's not dextrose.
- Daily U&Es – fluid titrated.
- Antiemetics – may need ondansetron.
- Support and reassurance.
- Thiamine.
- Steroids.
- Enteral, TPN.
- If intractable, consider TOP.

C

- Due deficiency in vitamin B_1.
- Diplopia, sixth-nerve palsy, nystagmus, ataxia confusion.
- Prevention – give thiamine prophylactically and avoid dextrose solutions.

Suggested answer

A

Appropriate investigations include the following: urea and electrolytes, as hypokalaemia, hyponatraemia and low serum urea are common (1); full blood count, as raised haematocrit is likely (1); liver function tests, as these are abnormal in up to 50% of cases (1); urinalysis, as ketonuria commonly occurs due to the patient metabolizing fat (1); and mid-stream specimen of urine, to exclude urinary tract infection as a cause of vomiting in pregnancy (1). About two-thirds of patients have abnormal thyroid function tests, and these do not require treatment, as resolution occurs when the hyperemesis improves (1).

An ultrasound scan is essential for dating of the pregnancy, as well as for diagnosing multiple pregnancy and excluding hydatidiform mole, both of which are more common in patients with hyperemesis (1).

B

The mainstay of management is adequate and appropriate fluid and electrolyte replacement (1). Normal saline [sodium chloride 0.9%; 150 mmol/l Na^+] or Hartmann's solution [sodium chloride 0.6%; 131 mmol/l Na^+] is recommended, and potassium chloride can be added to the infusion bag as required (1). [5% dextrose saline solution and 10% dextrose solutions are dangerous, as there is a risk of the patient developing Wernicke's encephalopathy with the use of these infusions. Double-strength saline is also contraindicated, as this may correct the hyponatraemia too rapidly and cause central pontine myelinolysis.] Initially, daily urea and electrolyte measurements should be performed, permitting appropriate adaptation and titration of fluid and electrolyte regimes (1). Antiemetics should be prescribed and given regularly, rather than on 'as required' basis, until vomiting and nausea are under control. Suitable agents include cyclizine [50 mg t.d.s., orally, intramuscularly or intravenously], metoclopramide [10 mg t.d.s., orally, intramuscularly or intravenously] or prochlorperazine [5 mg orally t.d.s.; 12.5 mg t.d.s., intramuscularly or intravenously] (1). Should these agents fail to control the vomiting, ondansetron [8 mg b.d. orally or 4–8 mg b.d. slowly intravenously], a highly selective 5-HT_3 antagonist, may safely be used (although it is not licensed in pregnancy) (1).

This woman should be given lots of emotional support and reassurance (1). Thiamine (vitamin B_1) supplementation should be given. If the patient is unable to tolerate oral thiamine hydrochloride [50 mg t.d.s.], an infusion of thiamine [100 mg diluted in 100 ml of normal saline], should be given over 30 minutes to reduce the risk of Wernicke's encephalopathy. Intravenous treatment is required only once weekly (1). In cases of protracted hyperemesis, oral prednisolone [50 mg daily in divided doses] or intravenous hydrocortisone [100 mg b.d.] often results in a dramatic resolution of symptoms (1). In very severe cases of hyperemesis, enteral or total parenteral nutrition (TPN) may be required. This should be administered in conjunction with advice from a senior pharmacist, as careful monitoring is necessary (1). [Thiamine supplementation is essential, as TPN has high concentrations of glucose.]

If the hyperemesis is intractable, and the patient is unable to cope and fails to respond to the above measures, then sensitive exploration of termination of her pregnancy may be considered (1). [It is very unusual that hyperemesis is so severe that termination is necessary.]

C

Wernicke's encephalopathy is caused by a deficiency in vitamin B_1 (thiamine). Clinical features include diplopia, abnormal ocular movements, including sixth-nerve palsy [lateral rectus muscle], nystagmus, ataxia and confusion (1). [Features on magnetic resonance imaging are symmetrical lesions around the aqueduct and fourth ventricle.] Prophylactic administration of thiamine to patients with hyperemesis gravidarum and not giving intravenous fluids containing dextrose can prevent Wernicke's encephalopathy (2).

Further reading

Crocker SG. MRCOG part II model essay answer. *Current Obstetrics and Gynaecology* 2005; 15: 422–3.

Nelson-Piercy C. Gastrointestinal disease. In: *Handbook of Obstetric Medicine* (3rd edition). London: Informa Healthcare, 2006: 218–26.

2.2.2.4

A 54-year-old woman taking combined hormone replacement therapy (HRT) for three years to relieve vasomotor symptoms attends the gynaecological outpatient clinic, concerned about the risks of continuing on HRT.

A Describe the risks to this patient of her taking HRT. (7 marks)

B Outline the advantages of HRT. (7 marks)

C How would you ensure she makes an informed choice? (6 marks)

Key words in the question

- 54-year-old, HRT, three years.
- Concerned, risks, HRT.
- Advantages, HRT.
- Informed choice.

Essay plan

A

● Risks – breast cancer, VTE, endometrial cancer, gall-bladder disease.

B

● Advantages – vasomotor symptoms, urogenital symptoms, sexuality, osteoporosis, colorectal cancer.

C

● Discuss advantages and disadvantages of HRT.
● Offer options – stop HRT. If flushes return consider progestogens alone, clonidine, SSRIs/NRSIs.
● Switch to ccHRT (no bleed and reduction endometrial cancer).
● Finally = patient's choice risk–benefit ratio.

Suggested answer

A

This patient has a small increase in the risk of breast cancer (about 3 cases extra per 1000) if she stays on combined hormone replacement therapy (HRT) for five years. The estimated increased risk of breast cancer is 2.3% per year. This risk disappears once HRT is stopped (3).

HRT increases the risk of venous thromboembolism (VTE). The greatest risk is in the first year of use. Since this patient has been on HRT for three years, her absolute risk is small. Approximately 2/1000 women over 50 who are not taking HRT get VTE, while this patient, as she is already on HRT, has about a twofold increased risk, i.e. 4/1000 (2).

This patient on combined HRT has a very low risk of endometrial cancer. However, combined continuous HRT carries no increased risk of endometrial cancer when compared to women taking no HRT, and therefore switching to a no-bleed preparation should be considered (1).

HRT increases this patient's risk of gall-bladder disease (1).

B

The advantages of HRT in this patient include relief of hot flushes and night sweats (2).

Symptoms of vaginal dryness, superficial dyspareunia, urinary frequency and urgency respond well to HRT (2).

HRT is very effective at reducing the risk of osteoporotic fractures but is not recommended as a first-line treatment for osteoporosis prevention, as the risks outweigh the benefits (2).

HRT reduces the risk of colorectal cancer by approximately one-third (1).

C

The patient should be informed of the advantages and disadvantages of taking HRT (see above). Since flushes seldom last longer than three to five years, she may wish to discontinue HRT and see if the flushes have stopped. There is no advantage to stopping HRT gradually or abruptly. Alternatively, she may feel reassured and continue on combined HRT (2).

If she stops HRT, urogenital symptoms may become apparent and topical oestrogen should be prescribed (1).

If her flushes return, she could try other pharmacological agents, e.g. norethisterone 5 mg daily, clonidine, or serotonin reuptake inhibitors or noradrenalin reuptake inhibitors, although the effect of these agents on reducing hot flushes may be short-lasting (1).

Another option is to switch the woman to continuous combined HRT, which will control the vasomotor symptoms, reduce her risk of endometrial cancer and may result in amenorrhoea (1).

Once all these options have been explained, the patient can make an informed choice, being fully aware of the risk/benefit ratio (1).

Further reading

Rees M. *Menopause for the MRCOG and Beyond.* London: RCOG Press, 2008.

Rees M, Purdie DW, eds. *Management of the Menopause: The Handbook* (4th edition). London: RSM Press, 2006.

Practice exam 3: Questions

Paper 1

2.3.1.1

A 30-year-old, insulin-dependent, diabetic woman attends the gynaecology clinic to discuss her plans for starting a family in the near future.

A What preconceptual advice should she be given? (7 marks)

B What are the specific risks associated with pregnancy in a diabetic mother? (7 marks)

C How should her antenatal care be planned? (6 marks)

2.3.1.2

A 40-year-old woman attends the antenatal booking clinic at 12 weeks' gestation. She is concerned about the possibility of having a Down syndrome baby and is requesting antenatal diagnosis.

A What options are available to her? Justify your advice. (6 marks)

B She decides to have an amniocentesis. How would you explain the procedure to her? (6 marks)

C How will you obtain her consent for the procedure? (8 marks)

2.3.1.3

You attend the labour ward for handover before a long day shift. You are informed that a primigravid woman in room 1 requires an instrumental delivery and are asked to attend immediately.

A What are the indications for operative vaginal delivery? (6 marks)

B What are the essential conditions for a safe operative delivery? (8 marks)

C Discuss the pros and cons of a forceps compared with a ventouse delivery? (6 marks)

2.3.1.4

A A 26-year-old, apparently healthy patient attends the antenatal booking clinic at 10 weeks' gestation. What specific questions would you ask her to screen for psychiatric disorder? (3 marks)

B A patient attends the gynaecological outpatient clinic. She gives a history of depression and has been stable on paroxetine for three years. She would like to start a family. Justify your advice. (11 marks)

C A 30-year-old woman with a known history of severe bipolar disorder books in the antenatal clinic at eight weeks' gestation. She has a very high risk of relapsing and needs to stay on lithium. What are the fetal risks of lithium in pregnancy? Outline an appropriate antenatal and peripartum plan. (6 marks)

Paper 2

2.3.2.1

A Outline the components of hormone replacement therapy (HRT). (3 marks)

B Describe three routes of administration and one potential advantage and disadvantage of each delivery system. (6 marks)

C How would you counsel a patient who wishes to switch from sequential to continuous combined HRT? (5 marks)

D What strategies would you use to reduce persistent oestrogenic side effects; persistent progestogenic side effects? (6 marks)

2.3.2.2

A Describe the steps involved in the audit cycle. (6 marks)

B How would you demonstrate that your surgical outcomes from any procedure are at an acceptable standard? Describe how you would set up such a review, using abdominal hysterectomy as an example. (14 marks)

2.3.2.3

A fit, 70-year-old, sexually active woman presents to your gynaecology clinic complaining of prolapse 25 years after hysterectomy for menorrhagia.

A Outline the initial assessment of this woman. (3 marks)

B Discuss the surgical options for vault prolapse. (6 marks)

C Discuss the outcomes and complications of the procedures identified in B. (11 marks)

2.3.2.4

A 24-year-old, nulliparous woman attends the early-pregnancy assessment unit (EPAU) with eight weeks of amenorrhoea, a positive pregnancy test and mild vaginal bleeding. An ultrasound scan (USS) is suggestive of molar pregnancy with no fetus.

A How would you explain this USS finding to the patient? (3 marks)

B What is the appropriate initial management of this case? (6 marks)

C What advice should the patient receive after treatment? (11 marks)

Practice exam 3: Answers

Paper 1

2.3.1.1

A 30-year-old, insulin-dependent, diabetic woman attends the gynaecology clinic to discuss her plans for starting a family in the near future.

A What preconceptual advice should she be given? (7 marks)

B What are the specific risks associated with pregnancy in a diabetic mother? (7 marks)

C How should her antenatal care be planned? (6 marks)

Key words in the question

- Diabetic, preconceptual advice.
- Specific risks, pregnancy.
- Antenatal care, planned.

Essay plan

A

- Good glycaemic control before pregnancy.
- Diabetologist referral to review medication.
- Folic acid supplement.

B

- Fetal risks.
- Maternal risks.

C

- Medical antenatal clinic.
- Good glycaemic control.
- Check for congenital malformations.
- Renal and retinal assessments.
- Appropriate fetal biometry.

Suggested answer

A

She should be informed of the importance of good glycaemic control prior to pregnancy and therefore unplanned pregnancy should be avoided (1). Strict glycaemic control both before and during pregnancy decreases the risk of congenital malformations, miscarriages, stillbirths and neonatal deaths (1). HbA1c of <6.1% is ideal. If the level is >10%, pregnancy should be avoided until better glycaemic control is achieved. Increasing the frequency of self-monitoring of her glucose levels will facilitate this (1).

A referral should be made to a diabetologist to review all her medication and to optimize her insulin regime (1). Baseline retinal (fundoscopy) and renal (urea and electrolytes) assessments are also performed to check for diabetic retinopathy and nephropathy (1).

If the patient is overweight, she should be advised to lose weight. A body mass index of 27 kg/m^2 or less is recommended (1). She should be advised to take folic acid 5 mg per day to decrease the risk of neural tube defects (1).

B

A pregnancy in a diabetic mother has increased fetal and maternal risks.

There is a 4–10-fold increase in congenital malformations, especially cardiac and neural tube defects (1). The perinatal mortality rate is also increased fourfold (1). Preterm delivery is five times more likely in a diabetic mother (1). The risk of shoulder dystocia and Erb's palsy are also increased, due to the associated macrosomia (1).

A diabetic pregnancy is more likely to be complicated by pre-eclampsia and polyhydramnios (1). Two out of every three diabetic women are delivered by caesarean section (1). Diabetic retinopathy and/or nephropathy may deteriorate during pregnancy (1).

C

A multidisciplinary team in the medical antenatal clinic should manage antenatal care of a diabetic woman (1).

At booking, an accurate dating scan is performed and a detailed anomaly scan is organized for 18–20 weeks' gestation (1).

A baseline HbA1c test is arranged. Antenatal appointments with the joint team should be offered every two weeks to monitor her glycaemic control. It is normal for increasing doses of insulin to be required as pregnancy progresses. Increased self-monitoring with fasting and one-hour post-meal blood glucose levels is advised (2).

A retinal assessment is performed at booking and at 28 weeks. An additional check is performed at 16–20 weeks if any diabetic retinopathy is found at booking. Renal assessment (urea and electrolytes) should also be arranged at the booking visit (1).

Ultrasound monitoring of fetal growth and amniotic fluid volume should be performed every four weeks from 28–36 weeks. The frequency may need to be increased if there are concerns about intrauterine growth restriction (1).

Further reading

Confidential Enquiry into Maternal and Child Health. *Pregnancy in Women with Type I and Type II Diabetes in 2002–03, England, Wales and Northern Ireland.* London: CEMACH, 2005.

2.3.1.2

A 40-year-old woman attends the antenatal booking clinic at 12 weeks' gestation. She is concerned about the possibility of having a Down syndrome baby and is requesting antenatal diagnosis.

A What options are available to her? Justify your advice. (6 marks)

B She decides to have an amniocentesis. How would you explain the procedure to her? (6 marks)

C How will you obtain her consent for the procedure? (8 marks)

Key words in the question

- 40-year-old, 12 weeks' gestation, Down syndrome, antenatal diagnosis.
- Options, justify.
- Amniocentesis, explain the procedure.
- Consent.

Essay plan

A
- Amniocentesis and chorionic villus sampling.

B
- Steps of the procedure.

C
- Explain procedure and reason for performing it.
- Procedure-related risks.

Suggested answer

A

The options available for definitive antenatal diagnosis are chorionic villus sampling (CVS) or amniocentesis (1). The recommended gestation for performing CVS is between 10 and 13 weeks and for amniocentesis after 15 completed weeks of gestation (1). Amniocentesis before 14 weeks is associated with significantly increased fetal loss and an increased incidence of fetal talipes (1). As she is at 12 weeks, CVS is an option. The risk of miscarriage with this procedure is 3% higher than with amniocentesis (1). The rate of miscarriage with amniocentesis after 15 weeks is quoted at 1% and with a skilled operator may be even less (1). Therefore, a reasonable option would be to undergo amniocentesis after 15 weeks' gestation (1).

B

I would inform the patient that an amniocentesis involves removing amniotic fluid from around the baby and sending the sample for chromosomal analysis (1). The abdominal wall is cleaned with antiseptic and an ultrasound scan is performed to identify the placental site and the deepest pool of amniotic fluid (1). Typically, a 20-gauge needle, which has a width of 0.9 mm, is introduced into the uterine cavity via the mother's abdominal wall, with direct ultrasound control and continuous needle-tip visualization (1). I would explain to the woman that this decreases the risk of fetal or maternal trauma and also decreases the risk of obtaining a blood-stained sample (1) [incidence of bloody tap decreased from 2.4% to 0.8%]. Local anaesthetic is not required, as the amniocentesis needle prick feels similar to having a blood test (1). If the woman is rhesus negative she will require administration of anti-D immunoglobulin (1).

C

The consent whether verbal or written should be documented in the notes and supported with written information (leaflets) (1). The reason for performing the procedure (higher risk of Down syndrome at age 40) should be explained to her (1). The procedure-related risks that require discussion with this patient are failure to obtain a sample of amniotic fluid, a bloody tap (as this hampers amniocyte culture), a miscarriage rate of 1%, fetal trauma or maternal bowel injury (though both are very rare), chorioamnionitis and failure of cell culture in the laboratory. The procedure causes mild discomfort at the needle site (4). The patient should be given contact details in case of any complications and should be given an idea of how long the result will take and how she will be informed (2). [The result is usually available in 48 hours.]

Further reading

Royal College of Obstetricians and Gynaecologists. *Amniocentesis and Chorionic Villus Sampling.* Green-Top Guideline No. 8. London: RCOG, January 2005.

2.3.1.3

You attend the labour ward for handover before a long day shift. You are informed that a primigravid woman in room 1 requires an instrumental delivery and are asked to attend immediately.

A What are the indications for operative vaginal delivery? (6 marks)
B What are the essential conditions for a safe operative delivery? (8 marks)
C Discuss the pros and cons of a forceps compared with a ventouse delivery? (6 marks)

Key words in the question

- Indications, operative vaginal delivery.
- Essential conditions, safe operative delivery.
- Pros and cons, forceps, ventouse.

Essay plan

A
- Fetal and maternal.

B
- Experienced operator.
- Abdominal examination.
- Vaginal examination – A, B, C = analgesia, bladder empty and cervix fully dilated.
- Availability of trained person in neonatal resuscitation.

C
- Ventouse – less maternal trauma.
- Ventouse – more cephalhaematoma, retinal haemorrhage and maternal worries regarding the baby.

Suggested answer

A

The indications for operative delivery can be either fetal or maternal. The fetal reason for an operative delivery is presumed or known fetal compromise.

Maternal reasons can be subdivided into medical indications and intrapartum problems (2).

Medical indications include those where a Valsalva manoeuvre is not advisable. Such conditions include some cardiac disease (class III/IV), hypertensive crises, cerebral vascular disease, uncorrected cerebral vascular malformations, myasthenia gravis and spinal cord injury (2).

Intrapartum maternal problems include a lack of progress in the second stage (active and passive) in a nulliparous woman, of three hours with regional analgesia or two hours without. In a multiparous woman these times are reduced to two hours with regional analgesia and one hour without. Other indications include maternal exhaustion and intrapartum medical conditions such as eclampsia (2).

B

Safe operative vaginal delivery requires an accoucher who is experienced in the type of delivery proposed, able to assess the clinical situation and able to communicate clearly with the woman (1).

A full examination of the woman is necessary. The operator confirms that the fetal head is less than one-fifth palpable per abdomen. On vaginal examination the vertex must be presenting and the cervix fully dilated, with the membranes ruptured. The exact position of the fetal head must be determined in order for the correct instrument to be selected and placed appropriately. The pelvis should be deemed adequate for the delivery. Informed consent (verbal) must be obtained from the patient and aseptic precautions taken. Adequate analgesia is required and this may be either regional or pudendal block. The maternal bladder must be emptied, and if a catheter has been in situ, this should be removed or the balloon should be deflated (5).

Adequate back-up personnel and facilities must be available, and anticipation of other complications associated with operative delivery, e.g. shoulder dystocia, should be borne in mind. Personnel who are trained in neonatal resuscitation must be available (2).

C

When compared with a forceps delivery, the ventouse is less likely to be associated with significant maternal perineal and vaginal trauma. It is more likely to be associated with cephalhaematoma, retinal haemorrhage and significant maternal worries about the baby. It is also more likely to fail at achieving vaginal delivery. There is no difference in the rate of conversion to caesarean section, low Apgar scores at five minutes, or the requirement for phototherapy for the baby (6).

Further reading

Royal College of Obstetricians and Gynaecologists. *Operative Vaginal Delivery*. Green-Top Guideline No. 26. London: RCOG, October 2005.

3

2.3.1.4

A   A 26-year-old, apparently healthy patient attends the antenatal booking clinic at 10 weeks' gestation. What specific questions would you ask her to screen for psychiatric disorder? (3 marks)

B   A patient attends the gynaecological outpatient clinic. She gives a history of depression and has been stable on paroxetine for three years. She would like to start a family. Justify your advice. (11 marks)

C   A 30-year-old woman with a known history of severe bipolar disorder books in the antenatal clinic at eight weeks' gestation. She has a very high risk of relapsing and needs to stay on lithium. What are the fetal risks of lithium in pregnancy? Outline an appropriate antenatal and peripartum plan. (6 marks)

Key words in the question

- Specific questions, screen, psychiatric disorder.
- History of depression, stable on paroxetine, three years, start a family, justify, advice.
- Severe bipolar disorder, risk of relapsing, stay on lithium, fetal risks, lithium, antenatal and peripartum plan.

Essay plan

A
- Past/present mental illness.
- Previous treatment.
- Family history.

B
- Acknowledge uncertainties, risks, risk–benefit analysis.
- Discontinue paroxetine gradually, monitor by GP or psychiatrist.
- If OK, try conceive on no treatment. If relapse, CBT $+/-$ antidepressant.
- TCADs. Breast-feeding, sertraline or TCADs.
- All associated with withdrawal in neonate – usually mild.

C
- Lithium – fetal heart defects and specifically Ebstein's anomaly.
- Serum levels four times weekly, weekly from 36 weeks, within 24 hours of delivery.
- Keep levels near lower end of therapeutic range.
- Hospital birth, avoid dehydration, risk of lithium toxicity.
- Avoid breast-feeding.
- Full neonatal examination.

Suggested answer

A

I would ask the woman questions about past or present severe mental illness (1), whether she has had previous treatment by a psychiatrist or specialist mental health team (1), and whether there is a family history of perinatal mental illness (1).

B

I would acknowledge the uncertainties surrounding the risks of using antidepressants in pregnancy (1). The risk−benefit analysis should be discussed, including the ability of the patient to cope with a pregnancy, risk of relapse, severity of previous depressive episodes and the woman's preference (2).

I would suggest to the woman that it would be best to discontinue the paroxetine because it is associated with fetal heart defects [especially ventricular septal defects] in the first trimester and persistent pulmonary hypertension in the neonate if it is taken after 20 weeks' gestation (1). Since she has been stable for more than six months (three years), I would recommend gradually reducing the dose of paroxetine, with monitoring of her mental health by her general practitioner or psychiatrist (1). Should she remain well, she could try to conceive without being on an antidepressant (1). If her depression recurs, she should have a trial of cognitive-behavioural therapy and/or be commenced on an antidepressant with fewer teratogenic effects than paroxetine (1). [The selective serotonin reuptake inhibitor (SSRI) with the lowest risk in pregnancy is fluoxetine.] A suitable alternative is a tricyclic antidepressant (TCAD), e.g. imipramine (1). If she wishes to breast-feed, she would be best served by taking imipramine or sertraline (a SSRI), as their concentrations are lower in breast milk than are other medications (1). However, tricyclic antidepressants are more likely to cause death than SSRIs if taken in overdose (1). All antidepressants carry a risk of withdrawal or toxicity in neonates, although in the vast majority of cases these effects are mild and self-limiting (1).

C

Lithium use in pregnancy is associated with fetal heart defects [risk increases from 8/1000 to 60/1000] and Ebstein's anomaly [risk increases from 1/20,000 to 10/20,000] (1).

Since lithium has a narrow therapeutic/toxic ratio, serum levels should be checked every four weeks, and then weekly from 36 weeks and within 24 hours of delivery (1). [The normal range is 0.4−1 mmol/l.] The dose of lithium should be adjusted to keep serum levels towards the lower end of the therapeutic range (1) [i.e. near 0.4 mmol/l]. She should deliver in hospital, and close monitoring of her fluid balance is essential to avoid dehydration and lithium toxicity (1). [Lithium levels should be measured in prolonged labour.] Breast-feeding is not recommended due to the risk of toxicity to the infant (1). The neonate should have a full paediatric assessment to exclude any anomalies, particularly cardiac ones (1).

Further reading

Antimanic drugs, section 4.2.3. *British National Formulary* (BNF), No. 52, March 2008: 200−1.

National Institute for Health and Clinical Excellence. *Antenatal and Postnatal Mental Health*. Clinical Guideline No. 45. London: NICE, February 2007 (reissued April 2007).

Paper 2

2.3.2.1

A Outline the components of hormone replacement therapy (HRT). (3 marks)

B Describe three routes of administration and one potential advantage and disadvantage of each delivery system. (6 marks)

C How would you counsel a patient who wishes to switch from sequential to continuous combined HRT? (5 marks)

D What strategies would you use to reduce persistent oestrogenic side effects; persistent progestogenic side effects? (6 marks)

Key words in the question

- Components, HRT.
- Three routes of administration, advantage, disadvantage, each delivery system.
- Counsel, switch from sequential.
- Strategies, reduce, oestrogenic, progestogenic, side effects.

Essay plan

A
- Oestrogen for hysterectomized women, Oestrogen plus progestogen for non-hysterectomized patient. Progestogen cyclically or continuously. Tibolone and testosterone.

B
- Oral – easy to administer, compliance not guaranteed.
- Patch – avoids first-pass effect and mimics the natural route of oestrogen delivery in premenopausal women, skin reactions.
- Subcutaneous implant – compliance guaranteed, risk of tachyphylaxis.

C
- If >1 year since LMP or 54-year-old patient. ccHRT or tibolone.

D
- Oestrogenic – reduce dose, change oestrogen type, change route of delivery.
- Progestogenic – reduce dose, change progestogen type, change route of delivery, reduce duration/frequency of progestogen.

Suggested answer

A

Hormone replacement therapy (HRT) consists of oestrogen alone for hysterectomized women, or oestrogen and progestogen for the patient with an intact uterus. Progestogens are given cyclically or continuously. Progestogen can be administered for 10–14 days every four weeks, or for

14 days every 13 weeks, or every day. The first results in monthly bleeds, the second causes bleeding every three months, and the last causes amenorrhoea. Tibolone is a synthetic compound taken daily by postmenopausal women who desire amenorrhoea. It is therefore similar to the continuous combined HRT in that it treats vasomotor symptoms and prevents osteoporosis as well as causing no bleeding. Tibolone also contains androgen and can therefore improve libido. Testosterone implants may improve libido but not all women are responders (3).

B

Three routes of administration are oral, transdermal skin patches and subcutaneous implants (3).

Oral HRT is easy to administer but compliance is not guaranteed. Skin patches avoid the first-pass effect and mimic the natural route of oestrogen delivery of premenopausal women but the patches may cause skin irritation or reactions. The subcutaneous implant guarantees compliance but some patients get tachyphylaxis (3).

C

By definition a patient is postmenopausal if one year has elapsed since her last menstrual period. However, if the patient is on cyclical HRT, she may have commenced this prior to cessation of menstruation. Therefore a pragmatic approach is used — by age 54 about 80% of women are postmenopausal, and patients beyond this age can be commenced on continuous combined HRT (ccHRT). Should the patient have had six months of amenorrhoea prior to commencing cyclical HRT, she may be switched to ccHRT before age 54. Continuous combined HRT or tibolone induces endometrial atrophy, resulting in no bleeding. Continuous combined HRT is known to reduce the risk of developing endometrial cancer compared with sequential HRT. Spotting or irregular bleeding is common in the first three to six months of therapy and does not require investigation. If the bleeding persists beyond six months, becomes heavier or painful, or returns after a significant time of amenorrhoea, endometrial assessment is warranted. Unfortunately, some patients have persistent irregular bleeding and a normal uterus and may decide to recommence cyclical HRT (5).

D

Persistent oestrogenic side effects may be eliminated by reducing the dose of oestrogen, changing the oestrogen type (e.g. conjugated equine oestrogen to oestradiol), or altering the route of administration (e.g. oral, transdermal patch or vaginal ring) (2).

Persistent progestogenic side effects may be alleviated by changing the type of progestogen (e.g. from a 19-nortestosterone to a 17-hydroxyprogesterone compound) or reducing the dose, but it is important to give sufficient progestogen to protect the endometrium. Reducing the duration of progestogen from 14 to 10 days or utilizing long-cycle HRT where the patient ingests progestogen on only 14 days every three months may help. Changing the route of administration (e.g. to intrauterine or transdermal patches) may reduce unwanted symptoms (4).

Further reading

Rees M. *Menopause for the MRCOG and Beyond.* London: RCOG Press, 2008.

Rees M, Purdie DW, eds. *Management of the Menopause: The Handbook* (4th edition). London: RSM Press, 2006.

2.3.2.2

A Describe the steps involved in the audit cycle. (6 marks)

B How would you demonstrate that your surgical outcomes from any procedure are at an acceptable standard? Describe how you would set up such a review, using abdominal hysterectomy as an example. (14 marks)

Key words in the question

- Describe, audit cycle.
- Demonstrate, surgical outcomes, set up, a review, abdominal hysterectomy.

Essay plan

A Describe audit cycle – topic, standards, pro forma to obtain data, review data versus standard. If standards not met – action plan, repeat audit after defined timescale.

B Use audit. Using audit cycle, describe how a surgical review can be undertaken.

Suggested answer

A

Audit has five principal steps, which are commonly referred to as the audit cycle.

The first step is to select the topic to be reviewed (1).

The second is to identify an appropriate standard. This can be done by taking international, national, regional or local evidence-based results against which the local findings can be compared. Where there are no standards, a literature review may allow a standard to be set (2).

Third, a pro forma is designed to record local information. Comparison is made against the standard (1).

Fourth, where the standard is not met, change is implemented in order to improve care (1).

A specified time frame is set to allow the changes implemented to make a difference to the clinical practice reviewed. The fifth and final step is for the audit to be repeated, to determine whether care has improved (1).

B

I would demonstrate that my surgical outcomes are at an acceptable standard by conducting an audit, following the audit cycle (1).

In a review of my outcomes in women undergoing abdominal hysterectomy, involvement should be obtained from the local audit department, which allows for collection of case notes and the audit to be logged with the local hospital (1).

The standard should be set from national figures, in particular in relation to the length of procedure, intraoperative complications such as blood loss, length of stay and postoperative complications (including return to theatre, transfusion rates, wound infection rates, pelvic haematomas and readmission rates) (5).

A pro forma would have to be designed to permit the collection of all the information required. This would also facilitate analysis of the data obtained (2).

Local performance can then be compared against the standard and statistically assessed. This could be presented in the form of summary statistics (e.g. means, medians and percentages) (2).

Once the data have been analysed, areas of deficiency could be identified and changes in practice implemented (e.g. introduction of intraoperative antibiotics if the wound infection rate was high and antibiotics were not currently being given) (2).

The audit should be repeated after an appropriate interval to assess the impact of the change implemented (1).

Further reading

Royal College of Obstetricians and Gynaecologists. *Understanding Audit*. Clinical Governance Advice No. 5. London: RCOG, October 2003.

2.3.2.3

A fit, 70-year-old, sexually active woman presents to your gynaecology clinic complaining of prolapse 25 years after hysterectomy for menorrhagia.

A Outline the initial assessment of this woman. (3 marks)
B Discuss the surgical options for vault prolapse. (6 marks)
C Discuss the outcomes and complications of the procedures identified in B. (11 marks)

Key words in the question

- Sexually active, prolapse, after hysterectomy.
- Assessment.
- Surgical options for vault prolapse.
- Outcomes, complications.

Essay plan

A
- Assessment by history, examination and assessment tools.

B
- Main procedures – sacrospinous fixation, open and laparoscopic sacrocolpopexy.
- Anterior and posterior repair are inadequate operations. No evidence yet for newer procedures involving mesh.

C

- Outcomes and complications of sacrospinous fixation, open and laparoscopic sacrocolpopexy.

Suggested answer

A

Assessment of the woman should be comprehensive and objective. It should include a detailed history, including the use of validated quality-of-life scores to assess the impact on the patient's life (1).

An examination should be performed using standard quantifying tools, such as the Pelvic Organ Prolapse Quantification (POPQ). The presence of anterior and posterior defects should be noted, as these may need to be dealt with at the same time as any vault surgery (2).

B

Anterior and posterior vaginal wall repair with associated obliteration of the enterocele sac are inadequate treatment for vault prolapse (1).

Sacrospinous fixation, and laparoscopic and abdominal sacrocolpopexy are all effective in treating post-hysterectomy vault prolapse (3).

There is currently insufficient evidence to recommend intravaginal sling procedures, total mesh procedures or vault suspension to the anterior abdominal wall, although all these have been described and used in clinical practice (2).

C

Reoperation rates in abdominal sacrocolpopexy are approximately 13%, while in sacrospinous fixation they are approximately double, at 26% (2).

Laparoscopic sacrocolpopexy has been shown to be as effective as open abdominal sacrocolpopexy but requires a high level of laparoscopic expertise and can be associated with a longer operation time (2).

Sacrospinous fixation may have a higher failure rate but it is associated with lower postoperative morbidity (1).

Complications of abdominal sacrocolpopexy include blood transfusion, visceral injury to bladder and rectum, incisional hernia, mesh rejection and wound infection (3).

Complications of sacrospinous fixation include blood transfusion, bladder injury, rectovaginal haematoma and vaginal pain (3).

Further reading

Royal College of Obstetricians and Gynaecologists. *The Management of Post-Hysterectomy Vaginal Vault Prolapse.* Green-Top Guideline No. 46. London: RCOG, October 2007.

2.3.2.4

A 24-year-old, nulliparous woman attends the early-pregnancy assessment unit (EPAU) with eight weeks of amenorrhoea, a positive pregnancy test and mild vaginal bleeding. An ultrasound scan (USS) is suggestive of molar pregnancy with no fetus.

A How would you explain this USS finding to the patient? (3 marks)
B What is the appropriate initial management of this case? (6 marks)
C What advice should the patient receive after treatment? (11 marks)

Key words in the question

- Eight weeks, amenorrhoea, USS suggestive of molar pregnancy.
- Explain, USS finding, patient.
- Initial management.
- Advice.

Essay plan

A
- Not a normal pregnancy.
- Needs evacuation.
- Needs follow-up.

B
- ERPC.
- Avoid oxytocics.
- Histological diagnosis.

C
- Register with national centre.
- Contraceptive advice.
- Follow-up for at least six months.

Suggested answer

A

The patient should be informed that the ultrasound scan (USS) reveals that this is not an ongoing pregnancy and that a fetus has not been formed. There is an overgrowth of placental tissue in the womb, which requires removal under general anaesthetic (3).

B

The patient requires admission for evacuation of retained products of conception (ERPC), blood for determination of blood group, full blood count and baseline serum beta-human chorionic gonadotrophin (βhCG) level.

An experienced gynaecologist should perform the procedure, as there is a risk of haemorrhage at the time of evacuation (3).

Cervical ripening agents and oxytocics are avoided until after the products have been evacuated, unless the clinical need demands, as these have a potential risk of disseminating the molar tissue into the bloodstream (1).

The tissue is sent for urgent histological analysis to confirm the diagnosis of molar pregnancy and the histological type, as this influences the prognosis (2).

C

The patient should be advised to return to the hospital if she experiences heavy bleeding, as there is a risk of retained products or continued proliferation of trophoblastic tissue in up to 15% of complete molar pregnancies (2).

The gynaecologist registers the patient with the nearest national trophoblastic centre. The three UK centres are in Dundee, Sheffield and London (1).

The patient should be advised that she requires outpatient monitoring of blood and urine, which is arranged by the regional centre. It is imperative she understands the necessity of regular follow-up, as occasionally this condition may lead to cancer (2).

She should avoid pregnancy until six months after the βhCG levels have returned to normal (1).

The combined oral contraceptive pill should be used only after the βhCG levels return to normal, which in the majority of cases is within two to three months of evacuation.

The length of follow-up is between 6 and 24 months, depending on the rate of fall of the hormone level (3).

Recurrence risk of molar pregnancy is 1/55 and the patient should be informed that her βhCG levels must be checked six and eight weeks after any future pregnancy (2).

Further reading

Royal College of Obstetricians and Gynaecologists. *The Management of Gestational Trophoblastic Neoplasia*. Green-Top Guideline No. 38. London: RCOG, 2004.

Savage P. Molar pregnancy. *The Obstetrician and Gynaecologist* 2008; **10**: 3–8.

Practice exam 4: Questions

Paper 1

2.4.1.1

A Give five reasons why a low-risk woman in labour might be commenced on continuous electronic fetal monitoring (EFM). (5 marks)

B What four fetal features are assessed when interpreting a cardiotocogram (CTG)? Describe how each of these features may be classified when interpreting a CTG. (12 marks)

C What is a pathological CTG? (1 mark)

D You perform a fetal blood sample (FBS) on the basis of a pathological CTG and the result shows a pH of 7.22. Outline your plan of management. (2 marks)

2.4.1.2

A 34-year-old, primigravid woman, with a body mass index (BMI) of $25 \, \text{kg}/\text{m}^2$ and no other medical problems, presents at 30 weeks' gestation with a painful left leg. It is swollen and slightly mottled in appearance.

A What will be the initial management? (6 marks)

B The diagnosis is subsequently confirmed to be a venous thromboembolism (VTE) occluding the left external iliac vein. Discuss her antenatal management. (6 marks)

C How should her labour and postpartum period be managed? (8 marks)

2.4.1.3

A woman is brought to the labour ward with severe pre-eclampsia at 38 weeks' gestation.

A Define severe pre-eclampsia. (2 marks)

B What are the clinical features of severe pre-eclampsia? (5 marks)

C Outline your further management over the next 24 hours. (13 marks)

2.4.1.4

A 31-year-old Jehovah's Witness patient with a history of anaemia attends the antenatal clinic for booking at 11 weeks' gestation.

A What steps would you take to optimize her pregnancy and delivery? (8 marks)

B In labour she requires an emergency caesarean section. How would you minimize the risk of haemorrhage? (5 marks)

C What is intraoperative cell salvage? Discuss its advantages and potential disadvantages. (7 marks)

Paper 2

2.4.2.1

A What are the properties of an ideal contraceptive? (4 marks)

B A 32-year-old woman with a body mass index of 36 kg/m^2 and who smokes 20 cigarettes a day attends for contraceptive advice. She has used the combined oral contraceptive pill in the past and would be happy to do so again. Counsel her. (10 marks)

C Give three advantages of long-acting reversible contraception (LARC) and three possible disadvantages. (6 marks)

2.4.2.2

Mrs Jones is a 38-year-old woman in the gynaecology clinic. She outlines to you a family history of ovarian and breast cancer. She asks for ovarian cancer screening.

A What are the two main genes associated with ovarian and breast cancer, where are they located, and how are they thought to cause cancer? (6 marks)

B Discuss the familial risk of ovarian cancer. Indicate how the genes referred to in answer A may increase a woman's cumulative risk of developing ovarian cancer. (5 marks)

C What ovarian cancer screening can be offered to Mrs Jones? (4 marks)

D Discuss the role of prophylactic surgery in this case. (5 marks)

2.4.2.3

A 25-year-old woman is admitted to the emergency gynaecology unit with lower abdominal pain and vomiting. She had an uneventful diagnostic laparoscopy for pelvic pain as a day case 36 hours ago.

A Excluding bowel injury, what differential diagnosis should be considered? (4 marks)

B What would make you suspect a bowel perforation? What should be the initial management of a suspected bowel perforation? (6 marks)

C How should this incident be managed after the bowel perforation has been treated? (4 marks)

D How can the risk of bowel injury at laparoscopy be reduced? (6 marks)

2.4.2.4

A previously healthy, nulliparous, 28-year-old woman presents with 11 months of amenorrhoea. Her level of follicle-stimulating hormone is 75 IU/l and that of luteinizing hormone is 58 IU/l.

A What is the likely diagnosis? Outline the possible causes of her problem and counsel her regarding this diagnosis. (9 marks)

B What other investigations are indicated? (5 marks)

C Review the treatment options. (6 marks)

Practice exam 4: Answers

Paper 1

2.4.1.1

A Give five reasons why a low-risk woman in labour might be commenced on continuous electronic fetal monitoring (EFM). (5 marks)

B What four fetal features are assessed when interpreting a cardiotocogram (CTG)? Describe how each of these features may be classified when interpreting a CTG. (12 marks)

C What is a pathological CTG? (1 mark)

D You perform a fetal blood sample (FBS) on the basis of a pathological CTG and the result shows a pH of 7.22. Outline your plan of management. (2 marks)

Key words in the question

- Five reasons, low risk, EFM.
- Four fetal features, classified, interpreting, CTG.
- Pathological CTG.
- FBS, pathological CTG, pH of 7.22, management.

Essay plan

A
- Meconium, fetal heart rate changes, decelerations, bleeding, oxytocin.

B
- Baseline heart rate, variability, decelerations, accelerations.
- Reassuring, non-reassuring and abnormal.

C
- Two or more non-reassuring features or one or more abnormal features

D
- Borderline result – repeat FBS in 30 minutes if CTG unchanged.

Suggested answer

A

Five reasons why a low-risk woman might be commenced on continuous electronic fetal monitoring (EFM) are the development of meconium-stained liquor (1), a fetal heart rate of less than 110 or greater than 160 beats per minute (bpm) (1), the presence of decelerations after a contraction (1), fresh bleeding in labour (1) and if oxytocin is commenced (1).

B

In interpreting a cardiotocogram (CTG), the four fetal features assessed are the baseline heart rate in beats per minute (bpm) (1), the variability (1), the presence or absence of decelerations (1) and the presence of accelerations (1).

These features are classified as reassuring, non-reassuring or abnormal (1).

The fetal heart rate is reassuring when it is between 110 and 160 bpm. It is non-reassuring if it is between 100 and 110 or 161 and 180 bpm. It is abnormal when it is under 100 or over 180 bpm, or a sinusoidal pattern is present for greater than 10 minutes (2). The variability is reassuring when it is greater than or equal to 5 bpm. It is non-reassuring if it is less than 5 bpm for between 40 and 90 minutes, and it is abnormal when it is less than 5 bpm for more than 90 minutes (2). Absence of decelerations is reassuring. If decelerations are present, they are non-reassuring if they are early or variable, or if there is a single prolonged deceleration of up to three minutes. In abnormal situations the decelerations are atypical or late, or a single prolonged deceleration lasts longer than three minutes (2). The presence of accelerations is reassuring but their absence is of uncertain significance (1).

C

A pathological CTG is one where the CTG features two or more of the non-reassuring categories or one or more of the abnormal categories (1).

D

This pH result is in the borderline category. With a pathological CTG and a borderline pH, my management would be to repeat the fetal blood sample in 30 minutes, provided the CTG remained pathological (2).

Further reading

National Institute for Health and Clinical Excellence. *Intrapartum Care*. Clinical Guideline No. 55. London: NICE, September 2007.

3 **2.4.1.2**

A 34-year-old, primigravid woman, with a body mass index (BMI) of 25 kg/m^2 and no other medical problems, presents at 30 weeks' gestation with a painful left leg. It is swollen and slightly mottled in appearance.

A What will be the initial management? (6 marks)

B The diagnosis is subsequently confirmed to be a venous thromboembolism (VTE) occluding the left external iliac vein. Discuss her antenatal management. (6 marks)

C How should her labour and postpartum period be managed? (8 marks)

Key words in the question

- 30 weeks' gestation, painful left leg.
- Initial management.
- Thromboembolism, left external iliac vein, antenatal management.
- Labour, postpartum, managed.

Essay plan

A

● Establish diagnosis and reassure patient.

B

● Plan treatment and combined medical antenatal care.

C

● Plan delivery and diagnose any thrombophilias. Advice for future pregnancies.

Suggested answer

A

From the history it is important to establish the duration of her symptoms, any leg pain or swelling, and any chest pain, haemoptysis or lower abdominal pain. Any relevant personal or family history of venous thromboembolism (VTE) and any risk factors for it should be established. Examination of both legs should be performed. The patient's anxiety and pain must be recognized (2).

If VTE is suspected, the patient should be started on twice-daily therapeutic doses of low-molecular-weight heparin (LMWH) (1).

The patient should be given advice about the use of above-knee compression stockings, and leg elevation for relief of pain and mobilization (1).

Compression duplex ultrasound of the leg needs to be arranged urgently (1).

D-dimer is not always helpful in pregnancy but full blood count and coagulation status should be checked, along with urea, electrolytes and liver function tests (1).

B

The patient requires anticoagulation with LMWH twice a day throughout her pregnancy. Ideally, she should be taught how to self-administer the heparin and advised to use compression stockings continuously. Early mobilization and good hydration should be encouraged and adequate analgesia provided (2).

She should be advised to return to the ward if she has any abdominal pain, chest pain or haemoptysis. She should also be advised to omit the next dose of her LMWH if she feels she may be contracting or if her membranes rupture (2).

Such patients should be managed in a combined medical/haematology antenatal clinic (1). [The measurement of anti-factor Xa levels is not recommended in this case.]

Involvement of a vascular surgeon or interventional radiologist regarding the insertion of an inferior vena cava filter may be considered (1).

C

LMWH should be stopped 24 hours prior to any planned delivery (1). Surgical intervention should be avoided if possible. If caesarean section is required, intraperitoneal and sub-rectus sheath drains should be placed, and the skin should be closed with intermittent sutures (1).

Epidural or spinal anaesthesia is contraindicated for 24 hours from the last injection of LMWH (1).

Prophylactic treatment should be recommenced three hours after delivery unless an epidural catheter is in situ, when LMWH should not be commenced until four hours after catheter removal. Anticoagulation should be continued for six months (2).

Compression stockings should be used for at least two years after thrombosis in order to avoid post-thrombotic leg syndrome (1).

Follow-up with a haematologist should be arranged to monitor the patient's anticoagulation status and subsequently investigate for thrombophilias (1).

Appropriate advice regarding contraception and future thromboprophylaxis should be given (1).

Further reading

Royal College of Obstetricians and Gynaecologists. *Thromboembolic Disease in Pregnancy and Puerperium: Acute Management.* Green-Top Guideline No. 28. London: RCOG, February 2007.

2.4.1.3

3 A woman is brought to the labour ward with severe pre-eclampsia at 38 weeks' gestation.

A Define severe pre-eclampsia. (2 marks)
B What are the clinical features of severe pre-eclampsia? (5 marks)
C Outline your further management over the next 24 hours. (13 marks)

Key words in the question

- Severe pre-eclampsia, 38 weeks' gestation.
- Define severe pre-eclampsia.
- Clinical features.
- Further management, 24 hours.

Essay plan

A
- Definition of severe pre-eclampsia.

B
- Clinical features.

C
- Further management to stabilize and treat patient.

Suggested answer

A

Severe pre-eclampsia is defined as severe hypertension, i.e. systolic blood pressure (BP) greater than or equal to 170 mmHg or diastolic BP greater than or equal to 110 mmHg on two occasions together with proteinuria of at least 1 g/litre (2).

B

Other features of severe pre-eclampsia include headache, visual disturbance, epigastric pain and vomiting, papilloedema, clonus, liver tenderness, abnormal liver enzymes, platelet count falling to below 100×10^6/litre and haemolysis. The last three make up the HELLP syndrome (5).

C

The management of this woman should be aimed at stabilizing her clinically and then delivering the baby at the optimal time for the mother (1).

Senior obstetric, midwifery and anaesthetic staff should be involved (1).

Antihypertensive treatment should be started in women with a systolic BP over 160 mmHg or a diastolic BP over 110 mmHg (1).

Labetalol orally or intravenously, nifedipine orally or intravenous hydralazine can be used (1).

Magnesium sulphate should be considered in this case of severe preeclampsia to reduce the risk of seizures. This is given as a loading dose of 4 g over 15 minutes and maintenance of 1 g per hour thereafter. The magnesium sulphate should be continued for 24 hours after delivery or the last seizure, whichever is later (3).

Fluid should be restricted to reduce the risk of fluid overload, which can cause pulmonary oedema, in the intrapartum and postpartum period. This should be restricted to 80 ml/hour or 1 ml/kg per hour (1).

The woman should be delivered once she is stabilized, with appropriate input from a consultant obstetrician and anaesthetist (1).

The mode of delivery should be determined after consideration of the fetal presentation, the condition of the fetus and cervical assessment. If vaginal delivery is unlikely in the timescale determined, then delivery by caesarean section should be undertaken (2).

The third stage should be managed with five units of intramuscular or slow intravenous oxytocin to prevent a hypertensive surge, which can occur with ergometrine (1).

Postnatally she should be transferred to a high-dependency unit, where treatment of her hypertension and observation for eclampsia can be continued, since almost half of convulsions occur after birth (1).

Further reading

Royal College of Obstetricians and Gynaecologists. *The Management of Severe Pre-eclampsia/Eclampsia*. Green-Top Guideline No. 10(A). London: RCOG, March 2006.

2.4.1.4

A 31-year-old Jehovah's Witness patient with a history of anaemia attends the antenatal clinic for booking at 11 weeks' gestation.

A What steps would you take to optimize her pregnancy and delivery? (8 marks)

B In labour she requires an emergency caesarean section. How would you minimize the risk of haemorrhage? (5 marks)

C What is intraoperative cell salvage? Discuss its advantages and potential disadvantages. (7 marks)

Key words in the question

- Jehovah's Witness, anaemia, booking.
- Optimize, pregnancy, delivery.
- Emergency caesarean section, minimize, risk haemorrhage.
- Intraoperative cell salvage, advantages, disadvantages, IOCS.

Essay plan

A

- Check Hb/ferritin. Treat with Fe if <10.5.
- If unresponsive parenteral Fe.
- JW – what blood products if any?
- Document plan in notes and sign advance directive.
- Consultant obstetric anaesthetist – cell salvage and rHuEPO.
- Identify risk factors for haemorrhage and active management of third stage of labour.

B

- Most experienced surgeon.
- Oxytocics.
- Carboprost.
- IOCS.

C

- Definition of IOCS.
- Advantages – higher postoperative Hb, reduce blood transfusion.
- Disadvantages – experienced personnel, risk of AFE, does not remove fetal blood cells.

Suggested answer

A

This patient should have her haemoglobin (Hb), red-cell indices and serum ferritin checked (1). If she is iron deficient or has Hb <10.5 g/dl, she should be commenced on oral iron therapy (1). Should she be unresponsive, intolerant or resistant to oral therapy, parenteral iron can be administered (1). It is essential to establish which blood products (if any) she will accept. There is variation among Jehovah's Witnesses – some accept platelets, coagulation factors and albumin, while others refuse all blood products (1). A clear plan of management, including the completion and copy of an advance directive, should be inserted in her hand-held maternity notes (1). It is prudent for the patient to see a consultant obstetric anaesthetist to discuss cell salvage (if available) and recombinant human erythropoietin (rHuEPO). Patients with refractory anaemia and risk factors for haemorrhage may be given a trial of rHuEPO (1). Risk factors for haemorrhage should be identified, e.g. high parity and multiple pregnancy, and emphasized to staff and patient (1). Active management of the third stage of labour minimizes blood loss (1).

B

The most experienced surgeon should perform the caesarean section in order to minimize blood loss (1). Appropriate use of ergometrine and oxytocin is essential (2). Carboprost 250 µg should be readily available if uterine atony develops, as this is refractory to oxytocics (1). [Eight doses at 15-minute intervals can be given intramuscularly.] If the patient accepts intraoperative cell salvage, she may be reinfused with her own red cells (1).

C

Intraoperative cell salvage (IOCS) involves suction of blood from the operative field and separating the red cells by centrifugation. The red cells are washed, filtered and available for retransfusion within a few minutes. Jehovah's Witnesses often accept the use of a cell saver provided it is 'in continuity' with their circulation (2).

The advantages of IOCS include a higher postoperative Hb level compared with control groups and a reduction in allogenic blood transfusion. Since Jehovah's Witnesses refuse blood transfusion, IOCS may be a life-saving procedure (2).

The potential disadvantages include the necessity for trained staff to have expertise and experience of IOCS (1). There is a theoretical risk of iatrogenic amniotic fluid embolism due to contamination of blood with amniotic fluid, but this has never been described in practice. The use of leucocyte depletion filters and commencing cell salvage after delivery of the baby are currently recommended to minimize this risk (1). IOCS does not remove fetal blood cells, and anti-D immunization (determined by Kleihauer test one hour after operation) is necessary for rhesus D-negative patients (1).

Further reading

Harmer M, Clyburn P, Collis R, eds. *Core Cases in Obstetric Anaesthesia*. London: Greenwich Medical Media, 2004.

Royal College of Obstetricians and Gynaecologists. *Blood Transfusion in Obstetrics*. Green-Top Guideline No. 47. London: RCOG, December 2007.

Paper 2

2.4.2.1

A What are the properties of an ideal contraceptive? (4 marks)

B A 32-year-old woman with a body mass index of 36 kg/m^2 and who smokes 20 cigarettes a day attends for contraceptive advice. She has used the combined oral contraceptive pill in the past and would be happy to do so again. Counsel her. (10 marks)

C Give three advantages of long-acting reversible contraception (LARC) and three possible disadvantages. (6 marks)

Key words in the question

- Properties, ideal contraceptive.
- 32-year-old, body mass index 36 kg/m^2, 20 cigarettes a day, contraceptive advice, counsel.
- Three advantages, LARC, three possible disadvantages.

Essay plan

A

- 100% effective, no side effects, easy to give and reverse, independent of intercourse and doctor.

B

- Not COCP as obesity and smoker.
- Options – POP, Mirena, Depo, Implanon, CuIUD.
- Advantages and disadvantages and information leaflets.
- Informed choice.

C

- LARC – less susceptible to incorrect usage, very effective contraception, cost-effective.
- Irregular bleeding, operation to insert and remove, long carry-over effect with Depo.

Suggested answer

A

The ideal contraceptive would be 100% effective, have no side effects or health risks, be easily administered, be completely and easily reversed, be independent of intercourse and be acquired over the counter (4).

B

This patient has at least two risk factors (obesity and smoking) and should not be prescribed the combined oral contraceptive pill (1). A body mass index of more than 35 kg/m^2 is associated with at least a fourfold increased risk of venous thromboembolism (VTE). Furthermore, smoking doubles the risk of VTE and is an arterial risk factor (2). I would advise this woman of the methods of contraception that do not increase the risk of VTE, e.g. progestogen-only pills (including Cerazette), Mirena, Depo-Provera, Implanon and copper intrauterine devices (CuIUDs) (5). I would explain the advantages and disadvantages of each method and give her written information (leaflets) about each option (1). Should she feel unable to reach a decision in clinic, I would offer her a further appointment to give her time to read the leaflets and decide which method is best for her so she can make an informed choice (1).

C

Three advantages of long-acting reversible contraception (LARC), e.g. Mirena, Implanon, Depo-Provera and CuIUDs, are that they are less susceptible to incorrect usage (1), they are very effective forms of contraception (1), and they are more cost-effective than the combined oral contraceptive pill because they reduce the chance of unplanned pregnancies (1). [Mirena, IUDs and Implanon are more cost-effective than Depo-Provera.]

Three disadvantages of LARC include the possibility of irregular bleeding with Mirena (in the first six months) and Implanon; persistent bleeding may occur with Depo-Provera and heavier menstrual blood loss is common with CuIUDs (1). A second disadvantage of LARC is that some, e.g. Mirena, Implanon and CuIUDs, require a small operation or outpatient procedure to insert and remove them (1). A third disadvantage specific to Depo-Provera is the potential long 'carry-over' effect following discontinuation – resumption of ovulation may take up to a year (1). [There is no delay in return of fertility with CuIUDs, Mirena or Implanon.]

Further reading

National Institute for Health and Clinical Excellence. *Long-Acting Reversible Contraception*. Clinical Guideline No. 30. London: NICE, October 2005.

Szarewski A. Choice of contraception. *Current Obstetrics and Gynaecology* 2006; **16**: 361–5.

2.4.2.2

Mrs Jones is a 38-year-old woman in the gynaecology clinic. She outlines to you a family history of ovarian and breast cancer. She asks for ovarian cancer screening.

A What are the two main genes associated with ovarian and breast cancer, where are they located, and how are they thought to cause cancer? (6 marks)

B Discuss the familial risk of ovarian cancer. Indicate how the genes referred to in answer A may increase a woman's cumulative risk of developing ovarian cancer. (5 marks)

C What ovarian cancer screening can be offered to Mrs Jones? (4 marks)

D Discuss the role of prophylactic surgery in this case. (5 marks)

Key words in the question

- 38-year-old, family history, ovarian and breast cancer.
- Genes, located, how, cause cancer.
- Familial risk, cumulative risk.
- Screening.
- Prophylactic surgery.

Essay plan

A
- *BRCA1* chromosome 17, *BRCA2* chromosome 13. Repair damaged DNA. Fixed mutations in other genes.

B
- Background family risk, risk with 1 and 2 first-degree relatives. Cumulative risk with *BRCA* genes.

C
- Screening not shown to reduce mortality. CA125 and TVS. UKFOCSS study. Genetic counselling and impact if positive.

D
- BSO reduces ovarian cancer and breast cancer but still risk of peritoneal cancer. Age for surgery depends on which gene.

Suggested answer

A

The two main genes associated with breast and ovarian cancers are *BRCA1* and *BRCA2*. BRCA stands for breast cancer (2).

BRCA1 is located on the long arm of chromosome 17 while *BRCA2* is located on the long arm of chromosome 13 (2).

Their function is to produce proteins which repair damaged DNA. Mutations in the genes cause the proteins to be abnormal and therefore the repair function is adversely affected (1).

It is thought that the defective *BRCA1* and *BRCA2* proteins are unable to help fix mutations that occur in other genes. These defects accumulate and may allow cells to grow and divide uncontrollably to form a tumour (1).

B

Women with no family history of ovarian cancer have a 1.5% lifetime risk. If there is one first-degree relative affected, then that risk rises to 5% (1). With two first-degree relatives affected it rises further, to 7% (1). Overall, approximately 5–10% of all cases of ovarian cancer are thought to be familial (1).

Having an identified *BRCA1* defect gives a woman a cumulative ovarian cancer risk of 39%, while a defect in the *BRCA2* gene gives a cumulative risk of 11%, both by age 70 (2).

C

There is no published evidence that ovarian cancer screening significantly reduces mortality. Such screening that is offered involves measurement of cancer antigen 125 (CA125) and transvaginal ultrasound scanning. There is currently a study UKFOCSS (United Kingdom Familial Ovarian Cancer Screening Study) which is looking at the screening question. It is expected to report in 2009 (2).

Identification of cancer susceptibility in a family by genetic counselling and then identification of a gene defect such as *BRCA1* or *BRCA2* may allow identification of cancer at an early stage or allow prophylactic surgery to be undertaken prior to cancer developing (2).

D

It has been shown that bilateral salpingo-oophorectomy in women with *BRCA1* and *BRCA2* mutations can reduce the risk of ovarian-associated cancers from 40% to around 1–2%. It can also reduce the risk of breast cancer by approximately 50%. A residual risk of primary peritoneal cancer will remain, at approximately 4% (2).

The patient's age at surgery depends on which gene mutation is present and whether the woman's family is complete. The risk of ovarian cancer in *BRCA1* mutations is low until the age of 30 and then rises steeply. For *BRCA2* the risk rises after age 40 (1).

In Mrs Jones' case (as she is 38 years of age) if she has a *BRCA* gene defect, prophylactic surgery in the form of a bilateral salpingo-oophorectomy would be a reasonable option provided that she is adequately counselled regarding the complications of surgery, premature menopause and the associated psychological issues (2).

Further reading

Devlin LA, Morrison PJ. Inherited gynaecological cancer syndromes. *The Obstetrician and Gynaecologist* 2008; **10**: 9–15.

Teale G. Ovarian cancer standards of care. In: Luesley D, Acheson N, eds. *Gynaecological Oncology for the MRCOG and Beyond*. London: RCOG Press, 2004: 97–108.

2.4.2.3

A 25-year-old woman is admitted to the emergency gynaecology unit with lower abdominal pain and vomiting. She had an uneventful diagnostic laparoscopy for pelvic pain as a day case 36 hours ago.

A Excluding bowel injury, what differential diagnosis should be considered? (4 marks)

B What would make you suspect a bowel perforation? What should be the initial management of a suspected bowel perforation? (6 marks)

C How should this incident be managed after the bowel perforation has been treated? (4 marks)

D How can the risk of bowel injury at laparoscopy be reduced? (6 marks)

Key words in the question

- Abdominal pain, vomiting, uneventful, diagnostic laparoscopy, 36 hours ago.
- Differential diagnosis.
- Suspect, bowel perforation, initial management.
- Managed, after, treated.
- Risk, bowel injury, laparoscopy, reduced.

Essay plan

A
- Consider postoperative complications.
- Consider other causes of pelvic pain.

B
- Abdominal tenderness and rigidity.
- Relevant history and nil by mouth.
- Relevant investigations.
- Surgical opinion.

C
- Thorough explanation of events to patient.
- Explain that this is recognized complication.
- Risk management report.

D
- Patient and technique selection.
- Adequate pneumoperitoneum.
- Use of sharp trocars and Verres needle.
- Verres should be left open on entry.
- Examination of entry site after trocar insertion.

Suggested answer

A

The differential diagnosis (excluding bowel injury) includes postoperative infection, e.g. intrauterine if the uterus was instrumented or portal entry site, urinary tract infection and intra-abdominal bleeding (2). Other causes not necessarily associated with her laparoscopy include appendicitis, gastroenteritis and ovarian accidents (1). She is unlikely to have early pregnancy complications, as she is likely to have had this excluded prior to her laparoscopy but these must be borne in mind (1).

B

A bowel perforation should be suspected in the presence of abdominal tenderness and rigidity. This may be associated with abdominal distension and absent or tinkling bowel sounds. A senior surgical opinion must be sought urgently (2).

The woman should be advised to stay nil by mouth and may need a nasogastric tube if the vomiting is excessive (1). Intravenous access should be established and blood taken for determination of urea and electrolytes, full blood count and serum amylase (1). A radiograph of the abdomen to check for gas under the diaphragm is not very helpful after laparoscopy, as there is always some carbon dioxide remaining after the surgery. A computerized tomography scan may be helpful where the diagnosis is doubtful (1). A patient with a bowel perforation needs urgent surgical intervention to treat the faecal peritonitis (1).

C

The patient should have been counselled prior to the laparoscopy that the procedure carries a risk of bowel injury (1) [0.6/1000]. A thorough and honest explanation of events must be given to the patient by a senior clinician as soon as she is able to take in the information (1). Appropriate follow-up must be arranged with the surgical and gynaecological team (1).

A risk management report must be made for this complication (1).

D

Adequate training of the surgeon and appropriate case selection will reduce surgical complications (1). If the patient has had previous peritonitis or a laparotomy, bowel adhesions must be suspected and an open laparoscopy (Hasson's technique) should be considered (1). The Verres needle and the trocars should be sharp to minimize the force used to insert them. This will reduce the risk of trauma (1). When inside the peritoneal cavity, excessive lateral movement of the Verres needle must not be performed, as that can exacerbate any bowel injury (1). Pneumoperitoneum should be maintained at 25 mmHg for inserting trocars so as to maintain a good distance from abdominal contents (1). On inserting the laparoscope, an inspection around the entry site of the trocars must be made to check for any injuries sustained during insertion (1).

Further reading

Lower A, Sutton C, Grudzinskas G. *Introduction to Gynaecological Endoscopy*. Oxford: Isis Medical Media, 1996: 71–98.

Royal College of Obstetricians and Gynaecologists. *Preventing Entry-Related Gynaecological Laparoscopic Injuries*. Green-Top Guideline No. 49. London: RCOG, May 2008.

2.4.2.4

A previously healthy, nulliparous, 28-year-old woman presents with 11 months of amenorrhoea. Her level of follicle-stimulating hormone is 75 IU/l and that of luteinizing hormone is 58 IU/l.

A   What is the likely diagnosis? Outline the possible causes of her problem and counsel her regarding this diagnosis. (9 marks)

B   What other investigations are indicated? (5 marks)

C   Review the treatment options. (6 marks)

Key words in the question

- Previously healthy, nulliparous.
- 28-year-old, 11 months, amenorrhoea.
- Follicle-stimulating hormone, 75 IU/l.

Essay plan

A   Causes of premature ovarian failure – chromosomal, autoimmune, enzyme deficiencies, FSH receptor gene polymorphism. Counsel.

B   TFTs, autoimmune screen, chromosome analysis. If necessary DEXA and ACTH stimulation test.

C   HRT or COCP $+/-$ testosterone. If desirous of pregnancy donor oocyte IVF.

Suggested answer

A

This woman has premature ovarian failure (POF) and often no cause is found (1). Where a cause can be identified it may be chromosomal abnormalities, e.g. Turner syndrome (45XO), Down syndrome (trisomy 21) and fragile X mutations. POF is also associated with autoimmune diseases, e.g. hypothyroidism, Addison's disease or diabetes mellitus. Enzyme deficiencies such as galactosaemia and very rarely follicle-stimulating hormone (FSH) receptor gene polymorphism can result in POF. Since this patient was previously healthy, secondary causes of POF such as bilateral oophorectomy or chemotherapy or radiotherapy are excluded. Occasionally mumps or tuberculosis can also cause POF (4).

The patient may find the diagnosis upsetting, especially as she has not yet had children. She should be informed that she likely has had an early menopause and this occurs in 1/1000 women before the age of 30. Although often infertile, spontaneous ovarian activity may occur, resulting in unscheduled bleeding, menstruation or even pregnancy. She should be offered support such as the Daisy Network, which provides psychological support. She needs long-term hormone replacement therapy (HRT) or the combined oral contraceptive pill (COCP) up until approximately age 52, to protect against osteoporosis and vasomotor symptoms. She can be reassured that there is no increased risk of breast cancer in taking HRT up to the average age of the menopause. Should she be desirous of a pregnancy, donor oocyte in vitro fertilization (IVF) is available (4).

B

Appropriate investigations for this patient are chromosomal analysis, thyroid function tests, fasting blood sugar, and autoimmune screen for polyendocrinopathy. If Addison's disease is suspected, the adrenocorticotrophic hormone stimulation test is performed. A dual X-ray absorptiometry scan may be performed to estimate bone mineral density (5).

C

Treatment includes adequate and sensitive counselling. The woman is offered HRT (oestrogen with cyclical progestogen) up until the age of 52 years. The dose of oestrogen may have to be increased if the patient experiences severe hot flushes. The COCP is also an option, and some patients prefer it because many of their peers use it (3).

Some women complain of lack of libido and/or persistent tiredness and may benefit from a testosterone implant or patch (1).

Donor oocyte IVF is the best option if this patient desires a pregnancy. Provided her karyotype is normal, the success rate is equivalent to that achieved in patients who undergo conventional IVF. The chance of a successful pregnancy is determined by the age of the donated oocyte rather than the woman's age (2).

Further reading

Rees M. *Menopause for the MRCOG and Beyond*. London: RCOG Press, 2008.

Rees M, Purdie DW, eds. *Management of the Menopause: The Handbook* (4th edition). London: RSM Press, 2006.

3

Practice exam 5: Questions

Paper 1

2.5.1.1

A The 2007 report from the Confidential Enquiry into Maternal and Child Health (CEMACH) sets out a list of 10 overarching recommendations. Identify five of these recommendations and explain why their implementation may help reduce maternal mortality. Do not use the Modified Early Obstetric Warning System (MEOWS) as one of your five examples. (15 marks)

B What are the principles behind the MEOWS and how might it help reduce maternal mortality? (5 marks)

2.5.1.2

You are the registrar on the labour ward and have just performed a ventouse delivery for fetal distress on a term baby.

A What is the Apgar score and how is it used? (8 marks)

B Describe how you would resuscitate a newborn baby. (Do not discuss the use of drugs.) (11 marks)

C When should resuscitation of the newborn be discontinued? (1 mark)

2.5.1.3

A 26-year-old patient at 39 weeks' gestation has significant contact with a five-year-old child who has chickenpox.

A What advice would you give the patient? (3 marks)

B If she is non-immune to chickenpox, outline appropriate management. (3 marks)

C The patient develops chickenpox. Discuss further management of this pregnancy and the subsequent monitoring of the newborn baby. (10 marks)

D What are the features of fetal varicella syndrome (FVS)? Why is it very unlikely this baby will have FVS? (4 marks)

2.5.1.4

A 24-year-old woman is seen at 15 weeks' gestation in the antenatal clinic. She is a known drug user.

A Give five maternal risks associated with drug misuse. (5 marks)

B Name three risks to the fetus when the mother uses heroin. (3 marks)

C Discuss neonatal narcotic abstinence syndrome (NAS). (6 marks)

D How would you manage this case antenatally? (6 marks)

Paper 2

2.5.2.1

A What factors are associated with an increased risk of ureteric injuries in obstetrical and gynaecological surgery and what can be undertaken to try to reduce this risk? (10 marks)

B Where are the common sites for ureteric injury? (4 marks)

C What postoperative symptoms and signs may suggest a ureteric injury? (6 marks)

2.5.2.2

A nulliparous girl attending the early-pregnancy assessment unit with right iliac fossa pain and seven weeks of amenorrhoea has just had an ultrasound scan that is suggestive of an ectopic pregnancy.

A What assessments of the patient need to be made in order to decide on her further management? (5 marks)

B Discuss the medical management of an ectopic pregnancy. (10 marks)

C What would be the prerequisites to allow an expectant management of ectopic pregnancy? (5 marks)

2.5.2.3

A 26-year-old, obese woman with polycystic ovarian syndrome (PCOS) attends the fertility clinic. She has been unable to conceive for two years due to anovulation. All other subfertility investigations are normal.

A Discuss how ovulation induction may be undertaken in this case. (11 marks)

B What are the risks for pregnancy in this woman? (9 marks)

2.5.2.4

A 46-year-old, otherwise fit and well woman is referred by her general practitioner with irregular heavy periods. On examination she has a bulky uterus. Oral progestogens have been unhelpful. She is very keen to avoid any hormonal treatment, including Mirena.

A What further details of her history are relevant? Using this information, outline initial management and medical treatment. (7 marks)

B Investigations show she has a uterine length of 12 cm with a 4 cm fibroid abutting the endometrial cavity. Considering her wishes, what non-medical treatment options does she have? (Do not discuss hysteroscopic resection.) (4 marks)

C Discuss the risks of hysteroscopic resection of fibroids. (9 marks)

Practice exam 5: Answers

Paper 1

2.5.1.1

A The 2007 report from the Confidential Enquiry into Maternal and Child Health (CEMACH) sets out a list of 10 overarching recommendations. Identify five of these recommendations and explain why their implementation may help reduce maternal mortality. Do not use the Modified Early Obstetric Warning System (MEOWS) as one of your five examples. (15 marks)

B What are the principles behind the MEOWS and how might it help reduce maternal mortality? (5 marks)

Key words in the question

- CEMACH, 10 overarching recommendations.
- Identify five, reduce maternal mortality.
- MEOWS, reduce maternal mortality.

Essay plan

A
- Preconception counselling, systolic BP >160 mmHg, CS and previous CS.
- Learn from serious untoward incidents, guidelines for obesity, sepsis and ectopic.

B
- Chart with parameters, detect life-threatening illnesses.
- Need action to reduce maternal mortality.

Suggested answer

A

The 10 priority recommendations include preconception counselling for patients with pre-existing serious medical or mental health problems [epilepsy, diabetes, cardiac disease, autoimmune disorders, obesity] which may be aggravated by pregnancy (1). This includes obesity and is especially relevant to women who are due to undergo fertility treatments. Implementation of this recommendation may help reduce maternal mortality, as many of the women who have died from pre-existing diseases did not receive pre-pregnancy counselling. Obese pregnant women with a body mass index of $>30 \text{ kg/m}^2$ are far more likely to die. They should be helped to lose weight prior to conception or any assisted reproductive technique (2).

   Another priority is that all pregnant women with a systolic blood pressure of 160 mmHg or more should be commenced on antihypertensive treatment (1). Should the overall clinical picture suggest rapid deterioration or the likelihood that severe hypertension will occur, consideration should be given to commencing antihypertensive treatment at lower blood pressures. In this report from the Confidential Enquiry the single most serious failing in patients with pre-eclampsia was inadequate treatment of systolic hypertension. Implementation of this recommendation may result in fewer deaths from cerebrovascular accident (2).

Mothers should be advised that caesarean section (CS) is not a risk-free procedure but may lead to problems in the current or future pregnancies (1). Women who have had a previous CS must have placental localization during pregnancy to exclude placenta praevia. If praevia is present, attempts should be made to identify placenta accreta and develop safe management strategies, hence reducing the risk of maternal death (2).

Another recommendation is that all clinical staff should learn from any critical events and serious untoward incidents occurring in their hospital (1). The plan to achieve this must be documented at the end of the incident report form. The lessons learnt should be actively disseminated to all clinical staff, risk managers and administrators (2).

Guidelines are urgently required for the management of the obese pregnant woman, sepsis in pregnancy, and pain and bleeding in early pregnancy (1). National guidelines are useful when there are unexplained variations in clinical practice, emerging problems and the recognition of persistent substandard care. The increase in maternal deaths in obese women is highlighted in this report. A guideline is needed, as, other than maternal risks, there are difficulties in prenatal diagnosis, an increased risk of gestational diabetes, an increased risk of requiring a CS and the challenges of anaesthesia and analgesia. Deaths from sepsis and ectopic pregnancy are often due to failure to recognize the problem promptly. Guidelines would help by addressing diagnostic issues in an evidence-based format (2).

[Other key recommendations

1. Ensure antenatal services are accessible and welcoming. Women should have a first booking visit and hand-held maternity record completed by 12 weeks' gestation.
2. If referred after 12 weeks, patients should be seen within 2 weeks.
3. All women who have not previously had a full medical examination in the UK require a full history and clinical assessment (usually by their general practitioner). Women from countries where genital mutilation is prominent, e.g. Sudan, Ethiopia or Somalia, should be sensitively asked about this during their pregnancy and a management plan for delivery agreed.
4. All staff must undertake regular documented and audited training for improvement of basic and advanced life support skills, as well as for the identification, initial management and referral for serious medical and mental health conditions, and the early recognition and management of severely ill pregnant women. Staff need to recognize their limitations and know when and whom to call for assistance.
5. Need to introduce the Modified Early Obstetric Warning System.]

B   The Modified Early Obstetric Warning System (MEOWS) is an early-warning scoring system that is modified for obstetric patients (1). It utilizes

CONTACT DOCTOR FOR EARLY INTERVENTION IF PATIENT TRIGGERS ONE RED OR TWO YELLOW SCORES AT ANY ONE TIME

	Date :																
	Time :																
Respiratory rate (breaths per min). Write rate in corresponding box	>30																>30
	21–30																21–30
	11–20																11–20
	0–10																0–10
Saturations (%)	90–100																90–100
	<90																<90
O₂ concentration (%)																	%
Temperature (°C)	39																39
	38																38
	37																37
	36																36
	35																35
Heart rate (bpm)	170																170
	160																160
	150																150
	140																140
	130																130
	120																120
	110																110
	100																100
	90																90
	80																80
	70																70
	60																60
	50																50
	40																40
Systolic blood pressure (mm Hg)	200																200
	190																190
	180																180
	170																170
	160																160
	150																150
	140																140
	130																130
	120																120
	110																110
	100																100
	90																90
	80																80
	70																70
	60																60
	50																50
Diastolic blood pressure (mm Hg)	130																130
	120																120
	110																110
	100																100
	90																90
	80																80
	70																70
	60																60
	50																50
	40																40
Passed urine	Y or N																Y or N
Lochia	Normal																Normal
	Heavy/Foul																Heavy/Foul
Proteinuria	<2+																<2+
	≥2+																≥2+
Liquor	Clear/Pink																Clear/Pink
	Green																Green
Neuro response	Alert																Alert
	Voice																Voice
	Pain/ Unresponsive																Pain/ Unresponsive
Pain score	2–3																2–3
	0–1																0–1
Nausea	YES																YES
	NO																NO
Looks unwell	YES																YES
	NO																NO
Total yellow scores																	
Total red scores																	

Figure 1 Stirling Royal Infirmary obstetric early warning chart. Reproduced with kind permission from Fiona McIlveney (and colleagues), Consultant Anaesthetist, Stirling Royal Infirmary, Stirling.

a chart for documenting parameters such as respiratory rate, temperature, heart rate, blood pressure, mental response, urine output, oxygen saturation, proteinuria and amniotic fluid consistency. The principle is that small changes in these variables combined will be seen sooner than will obvious changes in individual variables. Due to the changes in physiology of normal pregnancy, the scoring system requires modification, however (2). Such warning charts improve the detection of life-threatening illness (1). The recording of values on a chart is insufficient alone – it is the appropriate and prompt management and action that can alter the outcome, reducing the risk of maternal mortality (1).

[An example of a MEOWS chart can be seen in Figure 1, for information only. You will not be expected to include this chart in your answer.]

Further reading

Lewis G, ed. The Confidential Enquiry into Maternal and Child Health (CEMACH). *Saving Mothers' Lives: Reviewing Maternal Deaths to Make Motherhood Safer – 2003–2005.* The Seventh Report on Confidential Enquiries into Maternal Deaths in the United Kingdom. London: CEMACH, 2007.

4 2.5.1.2

You are the registrar on the labour ward and have just performed a ventouse delivery for fetal distress on a term baby.

A What is the Apgar score and how is it used? (8 marks)

B Describe how you would resuscitate a newborn baby. (Do not discuss the use of drugs.) (11 marks)

C When should resuscitation of the newborn be discontinued? (1 mark)

Key words in the question

- Registrar, ventouse, fetal distress, term baby.
- What, Apgar score, how, used.
- Resuscitate, newborn baby, not discuss, drugs.
- Resuscitation, discontinued.

Essay plan

A
- Heart rate, respiratory effort, muscle tone, reflex irritability, colour.
- Scored 0, 1, 2.

B
- ABC, dried, kept warm, call for help.
- Airway, five inflation breaths, ventilate at 30–40 per minute.
- If HR <60, chest compressions – 100 per minute.

C
- Senior decision – >10 min adequate resuscitation with no cardiac output.

Suggested answer

A

The Apgar score is a system used to assess the condition of the baby at birth (1). It uses five signs scored 0–2. The signs are heart rate, respiratory effort, muscle tone, reflex irritability and colour (1). The heart rate scores 0 if absent, 1 if below 100 beats per min (bpm) and 2 if above 100 bpm (1). The respiratory rate scores 0 if absent, 1 if slow and irregular and 2 if regular with crying (1). The muscle tone is 0 if the baby is limp, scores 1 if there is some flexion of the extremities and 2 if the baby is active (1). Reflex irritability scores 0 if there is no response, 1 if there is a grimace and 2 if there is vigorous crying or a cough (1). Colour scores 0 if the baby is pale, 1 if the body is pink with blue extremities and 2 if the baby is completely pink (1). The score is performed at one minute of age and repeated at five minutes, which allows an assessment of improvement in the baby (1).

B

The newborn baby is assessed for airway, breathing and circulation, in a similar way to the adult (1). The baby should be dried and kept warm (1). Paediatric help should be summoned (1). The airway should be checked and cleared. The baby's head is placed in the neutral position, and a chin lift and jaw thrust may be required to open the airway (1). Following the opening of the airway the lungs should be inflated with five inflation breaths over two or three seconds, using a bag and valve mask or continuous gas supply, a T-piece and mask (1). This displaces the fluid in the fetal lungs. This ventilation should continue at a rate of 30–40 per minute (1). After ventilation has been established, the heart rate may respond (1). If the heart rate remains below 60 bpm, chest compressions should be commenced (1). This is achieved by encircling the baby's chest with both hands so that the fingers are behind the baby and the thumbs are on the sternum, just below the level of the nipples (1). The chest should be compressed to one-third of its depth, at a rate of 100 per minute, with three chest compressions per ventilation (1). Once the heart rate rises above 60 bpm, chest compressions are discontinued (1).

C

A consultant in consultation with the parents and the resuscitation team should be the one to discontinue any resuscitation of the newborn. This is likely to occur in the presence of no cardiac output after more than 10 minutes of adequate resuscitation (1).

Further reading

ALSG. Resuscitation of the baby at birth. In: Grady K, Howell C, Cox C, eds. *Managing Obstetric Emergencies and Trauma: The MOET Course Manual* (2nd edition). London: RCOG Press, 2007: 69–81.

Baskett TF, Arulkumaran S. *Intrapartum Care for the MRCOG and Beyond*. London: RCOG Press, 2002: 175–84.

2.5.1.3

3 A 26-year-old patient at 39 weeks' gestation has significant contact with a five-year-old child who has chickenpox.

A What advice would you give the patient? (3 marks)

B If she is non-immune to chickenpox, outline appropriate management. (3 marks)

C The patient develops chickenpox. Discuss further management of this pregnancy and the subsequent monitoring of the newborn baby. (10 marks)

D What are the features of fetal varicella syndrome (FVS)? Why is it very unlikely that this baby will have FVS? (4 marks)

Key words in the question

- 39 weeks' gestation, significant contact, chickenpox.
- Advice, patient.
- Non-immune, appropriate management.
- Develops chickenpox, further management.
- Features, FVS.

Essay plan

A
- Ascertain if patient had chickenpox previously.
- Check serology.
- Reassure or VZIG.

B
- VZIG as soon as possible.
- Avoid susceptible individuals.
- If rash contact GP/midwife.

C
- GP, oral acyclovir, risks and benefits of acyclovir, avoid susceptible individuals.
- Urgent hospital referral if complications, nurse in isolation, multidisciplinary team.
- IV aciclovir and delay delivery if possible, epidural anaesthesia safest.
- Consider VZIG for baby, neonatal ophthalmic exam and blood for VZV IgM and IgG at 7 months.

D
- FVS = eye defects, neurological, limb hypoplasia. Very unlikely because maternal infection after 28 weeks.

Suggested answer

A

I would ascertain whether she had a previous history of chickenpox or shingles and confirm that she had significant contact with the child (1). I would arrange a blood test for serum varicella antibodies (1). Some 80–90% of women are immune. If this patient is immune, I would reassure her. If she is non-immune, she should be given varicella zoster immune globulin (VZIG) (1).

B

If she is non-immune, she should have VZIG as soon as possible (1). It is effective for up to 10 days following contact. The patient is potentially infectious from 8 to 28 days after the VZIG is administered, so she should avoid contact with other pregnant mothers and children who have not had chickenpox (1). She should notify her general practitioner (GP) or midwife if she gets a rash (1). [Should she be exposed again three or more weeks later and still be undelivered, she can be given a further dose of VZIG.]

C

If the woman develops chickenpox, she should inform her GP immediately. Oral aciclovir should be prescribed [800 mg q.d.s. for five days] if the patient presents within 24 hours of the onset of the rash (1). The woman should be informed of the risk and benefits of aciclovir (1). She should be advised to avoid contact with susceptible individuals, e.g. other pregnant women and infants, until the lesions have crusted over (1). [Chickenpox is infectious from two days before the rash appears until the lesions have crusted over. VZIG is of no use once chickenpox develops.]

If she develops chest or neurological symptoms, haemorrhagic rash or bleeding, she should be referred urgently to hospital (1). She should be nursed in isolation from babies and other susceptible individuals (1). She should be managed by a multidisciplinary team, e.g. obstetrician, virologist, neonatologist and, depending on the type and severity of the maternal illness, a respiratory physician or an intensive-care specialist (1). Intravenous aciclovir is given, and if possible delivery should be delayed until resolution of the rash. This permits transfer of protective antibodies from the mother to the fetus (1).

If anaesthesia is required for delivery, epidural is probably the safest method (1). After delivery, the baby should be given VZIG if the woman delivers within seven days of the onset of the rash. The infant should be monitored for signs of infection for four weeks (1). Neonatal ophthalmic examination should be performed and neonatal blood checked for varicella zoster virus (VZV) IgM antibody. At seven months a further sample should be sent to confirm VZV IgG antibody (1).

D

Fetal varicella syndrome (FVS) is characterized by one or more of eye defects (e.g. cataracts), neurological abnormalities (e.g. microcephaly), limb hypoplasia and skin scarring in a dermatomal distribution (3). This baby will not have FVS, as it does not occur in fetuses whose mothers become infected after 28 weeks' gestation (1). [This baby is at risk of varicella of the newborn – about 50% of neonates exposed to maternal varicella develop chickenpox even if VZIG has been administered.]

Further reading

Royal College of Obstetricians and Gynaecologists. *Chickenpox in Pregnancy*. Green-Top Guideline No. 13. London: RCOG, September 2007.

2.5.1.4

3 A 24-year-old woman is seen at 15 weeks' gestation in the antenatal clinic. She is a known drug user.

A Give five maternal risks associated with drug misuse. (5 marks)

B Name three risks to the fetus when the mother uses heroin. (3 marks)

C Discuss neonatal narcotic abstinence syndrome (NAS). (6 marks)

D How would you manage this case antenatally? (6 marks)

Key words in the question

- Five maternal risks, drug misuse.
- Three risks, fetus, heroin.
- Discuss, NAS.
- Manage, antenatally.

Essay plan

A
- Overdose, withdrawal.
- Nutrition.
- Needle problems.
- Infection locally.
- Hep B, C & HIV.

B
- Preterm delivery.
- SGA.
- Death.

C
- Develops 48 hours.
- CNS, GIT, respiratory, cry, poor feeding.
- Resolves in few days.
- Less pronounced in preterm babies.

D
- Multidisciplinary team.
- Non-judgemental care.
- Infection screening.
- Drug history.
- USS.
- Planned latter pregnancy, child protection.

Suggested answer

A

The risks include accidental overdose or sudden withdrawal, which can be associated with drugs of inconsistent purity (1). Women drug users often have poor nutrition and malabsorption, leading to iron, folate and vitamin deficiencies (1). If the woman uses needles, cellulitis, phlebitis and superficial thrombosis may develop (1). [Deep venous thrombosis can occur with femoral vein use.] Abscesses and, rarely, necrotizing fasciitis can occur with extravasation of the drug (1). [Systemic infection can develop following these local infections and this may present as septicaemia.] Hepatitis B and C and human immunodeficiency virus (HIV) infection are associated with intravenous drug use (1).

B

Heroin use in pregnancy can precipitate preterm delivery (1). It is also associated with babies who are small for gestational age (1). Fetal death can occur, particularly when fetal oxygen demands increase following withdrawal or abstinence (1). [There is also an association with acute placental infection, and there is a risk of vertical transmission of hepatitis B and C and HIV if present in the mother.]

C

Neonatal narcotic abstinence syndrome (NAS) usually develops within 48 hours of birth in the baby of a narcotic-dependent mother (1). It is characterized by central nervous system (CNS) hyperirritability, gastrointestinal dysfunction, respiratory distress, a high-pitched cry and poor feeding (3). It generally resolves within a few days, although the tremors may last for three months (1). The signs are less marked in the premature infant due to CNS immaturity (1).

D

The antenatal management of a woman with drug misuse should be multi-disciplinary, with input from obstetrics, midwifery, and psychosocial and addiction management (1). The woman should be given non-judgemental care, which will encourage her to attend the antenatal appointments (1). Infection screening, including hepatitis B and C and HIV, should be offered (1). A detailed drug history should be taken and conversion to methadone arranged if the woman takes street narcotics (1). Ultrasound scans every two weeks (from approximately 24 weeks' gestation) should be arranged to assess fetal growth and well-being (1). The woman, her partner and other key workers should meet towards the end of the pregnancy to plan management of the latter part of pregnancy and delivery, and the woman should be informed of the involvement of child protection agencies (1).

Further reading

Llewelyn RW. Substance abuse in pregnancy: the team approach to antenatal care. *The Obstetrician and Gynaecologist* 2000; **2**: 11–16.

Paper 2

2.5.2.1

A   What factors are associated with an increased risk of ureteric injuries in obstetrical and gynaecological surgery and what can be undertaken to try to reduce this risk? (10 marks)

B   Where are the common sites for ureteric injury? (4 marks)

C   What postoperative symptoms and signs may suggest a ureteric injury? (6 marks)

Key words in the question

- Factors, increased risk, ureteric injuries, reduce this risk.
- Common sites.
- Postoperative symptoms and signs.

Essay plan

A
- Factors associated with increased risk of trauma. Pre-op investigations e.g. IVU, intraoperative measures.

B
- Cardinal ligaments, infundibulopelvic ligaments, uterosacral. Commonest = lateral to uterine vessels.

C
- 50% have typical symptoms − flank pain and fever. Haematuria in some. Abnormal urinary leakage.

Suggested answer

A

The close attachment of the ureter to the peritoneum makes it particularly vulnerable during pelvic surgery. Certain factors have been recognized as increasing the risk. These include an enlarged uterus, previous pelvic surgery, ovarian tumours, endometriosis, pelvic adhesions, abnormal pelvic anatomy, coexistent bladder injury and massive intraoperative haemorrhage (4).

Preoperative and intraoperative measures can be taken to try to reduce the risk of ureteric injury. Investigations appropriate to the proposed operation should be undertaken; for example, an intravenous urogram (IVU) in cases where identifying the course of the ureter may be helpful prior to surgery, as in large fibroids (1).

Intraoperative measures include an appropriate operative approach, full examination of the pelvis and adequate exposure of the tissues. Direct visualization of the ureters in the pelvis has been shown to reduce the risk of ureteric injury (3).

Blind clamping should be avoided, as this has been shown to be the predominant cause of ureteric injury in obstetric procedures. Direct identification of any bleeding points is better than blind clamping (1).

Caution is necessary when using diathermy and laser at laparoscopic and open surgery, as long applications have been shown to be associated with ureteric injury (1).

B

Injuries to the ureters most frequently occur in the lower third (50%), followed by the upper third (30%) and the middle third (20%) (1).

The commonest site of injury is lateral to the uterine vessels. Other common areas include the area of the uterovesical junction close to the cardinal ligaments, the base of the infundibulopelvic ligament as the ureters cross the pelvic brim at the ovarian fossa, and at the level of the uterosacral ligament (3).

C

Postoperative symptoms of ureteric injury can be variable and only 50% of women present with typical symptoms (1).

The commonest symptoms are flank pain and fever (2).

Haematuria is present in about 70% of cases. Women may present with a retroperitoneal urinoma, which may be confirmed on ultrasound scan. Postoperative anuria should prompt urgent investigation, although this condition is uncommon. Urine leakage from anywhere other than the urethra should suggest the possibility of a fistula (3).

Further reading

Jha S, Coomarasamy A, Chan K. Ureteric injury in obstetric and gynaecological surgery. *The Obstetrician and Gynaecologist* 2004; 6: 203–8.

2.5.2.2

A nulliparous girl attending the early-pregnancy assessment unit with right iliac fossa pain and seven weeks of amenorrhoea has just had an ultrasound scan that is suggestive of an ectopic pregnancy.

A What assessments of the patient need to be made in order to decide on her further management? (5 marks)

B Discuss the medical management of an ectopic pregnancy. (10 marks)

C What would be the prerequisites to allow an expectant management of ectopic pregnancy? (5 marks)

Key words in the question

- Right iliac fossa pain, ultrasound, suggestive, ectopic pregnancy.
- Assessment, patient, further management.
- Discuss, medical management, ectopic pregnancy.
- Prerequisites, expectant management.

Essay plan

A
- History of pain.
- Haemodynamic stability.
- Serum βhCG level.
- Ultrasound findings.

B
- Identify patients suitable for this modality of treatment.
- Methotrexate intramuscular injection with serum βhCG follow-up.
- Inform patient about the importance of close follow-up.

C
- Stable and pain-free patient.
- Serum βhCG <1000 IU/l and ectopic mass <4 cm.
- Ability for close follow-up and urgent action.

Suggested answer

A

The patient should be asked about the duration and intensity of her pain (1). The presence of shoulder-tip pain or fainting may be suggestive of intraperitoneal bleeding (1). The haemodynamic state and any signs of an acute abdomen, e.g. rigidity or guarding, will determine the urgency and type of her treatment (1). Serial serum beta-human chorionic gonadotrophin (βhCG) levels should be checked to confirm the diagnosis and will help to decide on the modality of treatment (1). The ultrasound scan should be reviewed to establish the size of the adnexal mass, any sign of fetal heart pulsations within it, and whether there is free fluid in the pouch of Douglas (1).

B

The medical management of an ectopic pregnancy is more likely to be successful if the size of the adnexal mass is less than 4 cm, the serum βhCG level is less than 3000 IU/l, and there are no fetal heart pulsations seen on ultrasound (2). The patient must also be haemodynamically stable and relatively pain free (1). There should be no contraindication to the use of methotrexate and the patient should understand and agree to the importance of outpatient follow-up in this mode of treatment (2). A single intramuscular injection of methotrexate at a dose of 50 mg/m² is administered (1). Patients should be informed that they are likely to experience some 'separation pain' due to tubal abortion (1). If the pain becomes severe, the patient should attend the hospital urgently, as approximately 10% of cases require surgical intervention (1). Serum βhCG follow-up is arranged for days 4 and 7 and then weekly until resolution is complete. The level should fall by 15% between days 4 and 7. If this drop is not achieved, a second dose of methotrexate is required (1). Patients should be advised to avoid sexual intercourse during the time of the treatment and to use contraception for three months after, because of the potential teratogenic risk of methotrexate (1).

C

The prerequisite for allowing expectant management of ectopic pregnancy is a stable and pain-free patient (1). Serum βhCG levels should be less than

1000 IU/l and falling (1). The size of the ectopic mass should be less than 4 cm and there should be less than 100 ml of free fluid in the pelvis (2). The patient should be well informed about the necessity of close follow-up and must live within a reasonable distance of the hospital in order to attend quickly in an emergency (1).

Further reading

Royal College of Obstetricians and Gynaecologists. *The Management of Tubal Pregnancy*. Green-Top Guideline No. 21. London: RCOG, May 2004.

2.5.2.3

A 26-year-old, obese woman with polycystic ovarian syndrome (PCOS) attends the fertility clinic. She has been unable to conceive for two years due to anovulation. All other subfertility investigations are normal.

A Discuss how ovulation induction may be undertaken in this case. (11 marks)

B What are the risks for pregnancy in this woman? (9 marks)

Key words in the question

- 26-year-old, obese, PCOS.
- Discuss, ovulation induction.
- Risks for pregnancy.

Essay plan

A
- Weight reduction.
- Anti-oestrogen.
- Ovarian drilling.
- Metformin with or without anti-oestrogen.
- Gonadotrophins.

B
- Risks to mother – miscarriage, GDM, PET.
- Risks to fetus – SGA, preterm delivery, shoulder dystocia, neonatal admission.
- Ovulation induction – OHSS, multiple pregnancy.

Suggested answer

A

This woman should initially be advised to lose weight, as this improves both spontaneous and drug-induced ovulation (1). The first-line treatment should be with an anti-oestrogen, e.g. clomiphene citrate 50–100 mg, from days 2 to 6 of her menstrual cycle. If ovulation is achieved, the same dose should be continued until she conceives or for a maximum of 12 months (1). There is a 7–10% risk of multiple pregnancy and therefore follicular tracking monitoring with ultrasound is advised (1). Laparoscopic ovarian drilling is just as effective as gonadotrophins in achieving ovulation and does not carry any increased risk of multiple pregnancy (1). Since the recognition of insulin resistance in polycystic ovarian syndrome (PCOS), metformin has been used as an insulin-sensitizing agent. This ameliorates the hyperandrogenic state and can be used along with clomiphene in patients with a body mass index >25 kg/m^2, to increase the ovulation and pregnancy rates. However, metformin is not licensed for use in PCOS (2). If the above methods fail to achieve ovulation, gonadotrophins [human menopausal gonadotrophins, urinary follicle-stimulating hormone (FSH) or recombinant FSH] may be used (1). These are used intramuscularly, as success with subcutaneous pulsatile use in clomiphene-resistant PCOS patients is uncertain (1). In this group of patients, concomitant use of gonadotrophin-releasing hormone agonist is avoided, as it does not improve pregnancy rates and is associated with a higher risk of ovarian hyperstimulation syndrome (OHSS) (1). Ultrasound monitoring for follicle size and number should be an integral part of patient management during gonadotrophin therapy, as there is risk of OHSS (1%) and multiple pregnancy (35%) (2).

B

This woman has three risk factors that may adversely affect any pregnancy. They are PCOS, obesity and the fact that the patient has conceived via ovulation induction. Consequently, she has a higher risk of miscarriage (1). During pregnancy she is at an increased risk of developing gestational diabetes mellitus and its complications (1). She is also at risk of pre-eclampsia (1), preterm birth (1) and having a fetus small for gestational age (1). If her pregnancy occurs following ovulation induction, she has a 4% risk of OHSS (1), and a 10% risk of multiple pregnancy with clomiphene and an up to 20% risk with gonadotrophins (1). This woman's baby has a higher chance of admission to a neonatal unit (1). In addition, maternal obesity is associated with fetal macrosomia and shoulder dystocia (1).

Further reading

Balen A. The current understanding of polycystic ovary syndrome. *The Obstetrician and Gynaecologist* 2004; **6**: 66–74.

Boomsma CM, Fauser BC, Macklon NS. Pregnancy complications in women with polycystic ovarian syndrome. *Seminars in Reproductive Medicine* 2008; **26**: 72–84.

National Institute for Health and Clinical Excellence. *Fertility: Assessment and Treatment for People with Fertility Problems.* Clinical Guideline No. 11. London: NICE, February 2004.

2.5.2.4

A 46-year-old, otherwise fit and well woman is referred by her general practitioner with irregular heavy periods. On examination she has a bulky uterus. Oral progestogens have been unhelpful. She is very keen to avoid any hormonal treatment, including Mirena.

A What further details of her history are relevant? Using this information, outline initial management and medical treatment. (7 marks)

B Investigations show she has a uterine length of 12 cm with a 4 cm fibroid abutting the endometrial cavity. Considering her wishes, what non-medical treatment options does she have? (Do not discuss hysteroscopic resection.) (4 marks)

C Discuss the risks of hysteroscopic resection of fibroids. (9 marks)

Key words in the question

- 46-year-old, irregular heavy periods, progestogens, unhelpful, avoid, hormonal treatment.
- Further details, history, initial management, medical treatment.
- 4 cm fibroid, non-medical treatment options, not discuss hysteroscopic resection.
- Risks, hysteroscopic resection.

Essay plan

A
- Obstetric and gynaecology history.
- Endometrial sampling and ultrasound.
- Tranexamic acid, NSAIDs.

B
- Unsuitable for second-generation techniques.
- Uterine artery embolization.
- Myomectomy.
- Hysterectomy.

C
- Intraoperative.
- Postoperative.
- Delayed.

Suggested answer

A

History taking should establish the length and pattern of bleeding and its impact on the patient's quality of life (1). Any associated pain during or before her period and for how long the periods have been abnormal should be established (1). Other important information includes her obstetric history, whether she has completed her family, and her current method of contraception (1). Examination should establish the size of the uterus and any adnexal abnormality (1). As this woman is over 45 years of age with irregular bleeding, further assessment of the endometrium, to rule out hyperplasia or malignancy, should be performed (1). An ultrasound scan also needs to be arranged (1). Suitable initial treatments include tranexamic acid and non-steroidal anti-inflammatory drugs (NSAIDs) to reduce menstrual loss (1).

B

Since the fibroid is greater than 3 cm and the uterine length is 12 cm, she is unsuitable for any second-generation endometrial ablation techniques (1). The options available to her therefore are uterine artery embolization, myomectomy or a hysterectomy (3).

C

The intraoperative complications of this procedure include haemorrhage, perforation of the uterus and potential damage to intra-abdominal organs (2). Fluid overload can complicate the procedure, resulting in pulmonary and cerebral oedema, hyponatraemia, seizures, coma and death (2). Postoperative complications include infection, haematometra with cyclical pain and uterine synechiae (2). A late complication can be postablation pregnancy, which may be dangerous to mother and baby because of the poor quality of endometrium and synechiae (1). Fibroids or menorrhagia may recur (1). If an endometrial carcinoma develops after this procedure, it may be occult, delaying the diagnosis (1).

Further reading

Justin W, Ibraheim M, Bagtharia S, Haloob R. Current minimal access techniques in the treatment of heavy menstrual bleeding. *The Obstetrician and Gynaecologist* 2007; **9**: 223–32.

National Institute for Health and Clinical Excellence. *Heavy Menstrual Bleeding*. Clinical Guideline No. 44. London: NICE, January 2007.

Practice exam 6: Questions

Paper I

2.6.1.1

A 25-year-old epileptic woman attends the antenatal booking clinic at six weeks' gestation. She takes phenytoin and sodium valproate. She has had one convulsion in the past year, which occurred four months ago.

A What are the teratogenic effects of these drugs? (6 marks)

B How will you manage her antenatally? (8 marks)

C Outline postnatal and future management. (6 marks)

2.6.1.2

A primigravid patient 34 weeks' pregnant comes to see you in the antenatal clinic requesting a home birth.

A What is the approximate home birth rate in the UK? (I mark)

B What are the advantages of a planned home birth? (8 marks)

C What are the two commonest indications for transfer to hospital for a woman planning a home birth? (2 marks)

D Give three examples of the risks of delivering at home. (4 marks)

E What local arrangements must be in place to support home births? (5 marks)

2.6.1.3

A 26-year-old primigravida at 30 weeks' gestation presents to the antenatal clinic with widespread itching.

A Describe initial management. (6 marks)

B A diagnosis of obstetric cholestasis (OC) is made. How should the rest of her pregnancy be managed? (10 marks)

C How should she be managed in the postnatal period? (4 marks)

2.6.1.4

A What is female genital mutilation (FGM)? Outline the different types. (5 marks)

B A patient with FGM books for antenatal care at 12 weeks' gestation in her first pregnancy. Outline appropriate antenatal and delivery management. (7 marks)

C If this woman has type 3 FGM, what are the possible obstetric complications? (7 marks)

D Following delivery she requests reinfibulation. What would you do? (I mark)

Paper 2

2.6.2.1

Jane, a 15-year-old girl, attends a party and has unprotected sex with a 16-year-old, James, whom she knows from school. Jane comes from a strict Catholic background. She attends the accident and emergency department the next day requesting emergency contraception. You are the gynaecology doctor on call.

A Outline what further information you would need in order to counsel and treat this girl. (7 marks)

B Discuss the criteria, in relation to this case, which need to be met to deem someone less than 16 years of age 'Fraser ruling competent'. (4 marks)

C Would you do anything differently if Jane were aged 13 years or less? Is there an ethical dilemma to maintain confidentiality? (5 marks)

D The emergency contraception fails and Jane attends the outpatient clinic six weeks later requesting termination of pregnancy. She comes with her 17-year-old sister, who offers to sign the consent form for Jane, as their parents remain unaware of the pregnancy. What do you do? (4 marks)

2.6.2.2

A Outline the surgical options for the treatment of stress urinary incontinence (SUI). (5 marks)

B Using your answer to A, discuss the success rates and main complications for each procedure. (15 marks)

2.6.2.3

A 27-year-old, nulliparous woman is referred to the gynaecology outpatient department with symptoms strongly suggestive of endometriosis.

A What clinical features are typically associated with endometriosis? (6 marks)

B How can endometriosis be definitively diagnosed? (1 mark)

C Discuss the medical treatment options available if this patient has endometriosis-associated pain? (5 marks)

D What surgical options are available for treating endometriosis? (6 marks)

E If this patient has minimal–mild endometriosis and wishes to conceive, outline your management. (2 marks)

2.6.2.4

A 15-year-old girl presents with delayed pubertal development. Chromosomal investigations reveal Turner syndrome.

A Outline your principles of management. (8 marks)

B Justify your management through adolescence. (6 marks)

C Justify your management through adult life. (6 marks)

Practice exam 6: Answers

Paper 1

2.6.1.1

A 25-year-old epileptic woman attends the antenatal booking clinic at six weeks' gestation. She takes phenytoin and sodium valproate. She has had one convulsion in the past year, which occurred four months ago.

A What are the teratogenic effects of these drugs? (6 marks)
B How will you manage her antenatally? (8 marks)
C Outline postnatal and future management. (6 marks)

Key words in the question

- Epileptic, phenytoin, sodium valproate, convulsion, four months ago.
- Teratogenic effects, drugs.
- Manage, antenatally.
- Postnatal, future, management.

Essay plan

A
- Neural tube defect.
- Cardiac defects.
- Fetal anticonvulsant syndrome.

B
- Folic acid.
- Screening for abnormalities.
- Medical antenatal clinic with physician involvement.
- Vitamin K.

C
- Neonatal vitamin K.
- Advice on breast-feeding.
- Contraceptive advice.
- Referral to neurologist.

Suggested answer

A

The risks with sodium valproate are neural tube defects, congenital heart defects and hypospadias (2). Phenytoin is associated with congenital heart defects and orofacial clefts (2). Minor malformations (fetal anticonvulsant syndrome) associated with these drugs include dysmorphic features [low-set ears, broad nasal bridge and irregular teeth], hypertelorism, hypoplastic nails and distal digits (1). The risk of teratogenesis with one antiepileptic drug is 6–7% but increases to 15% when the woman is taking two drugs (1).

B

If she is not currently taking folic acid, she should be commenced on 5 mg folic acid daily throughout the pregnancy. This decreases the risk of neural tube defects and reduces the risk of folate-deficiency anaemia (1). She should be offered serum α-fetoprotein screening and a detailed ultrasound scan at 18–20 weeks (2). An additional scan at 22 weeks for cardiac defects may be offered if these are suspected (1). Monitoring of her drug levels is not required unless she has a seizure during pregnancy (1). She should be warned that there is an increased risk of seizures during pregnancy (1). She should preferably be managed in conjunction with a physician in a medical antenatal clinic, as her drug doses may need to be increased (1). As she takes an enzyme-inducing drug (phenytoin), I would prescribe daily vitamin K 10 mg orally for the last four weeks of pregnancy in order to reduce the risk of haemorrhagic disease of the newborn (1).

C

If her medication was increased during pregnancy, this can be gradually reduced during the puerperium to prepregnancy doses (1). The neonate should receive vitamin K (1 mg intramuscularly) (1). Breast-feeding should be encouraged, as the level of antiepileptic drugs secreted in breast milk is very low (1). The mother should be advised how to minimize the risk to the baby should she have a fit, e.g. bathing the baby in shallow water or with supervision (1).

Contraception should be discussed with the patient. If she takes the combined oral contraceptive pill, the dose of oestrogen will have to be 50 μg because of the hepatic enzyme-inducing effect of phenytoin. Higher doses of the progesterone-only pill will also be required. Depo-Provera is a good alternative (1). She should be referred to a neurologist for consideration of conversion to monotherapy before embarking on any future pregnancy (1).

Further reading

Adab N, Chadwick DW. Management of women with epilepsy during pregnancy. *The Obstetrician and Gynaecologist* 2006; 8; 20–5.
Nelson-Piercy C. Neurological problems. In: *Handbook of Obstetric Medicine* (3rd edition). London: Informa Healthcare, 2006: 156–79.

2.6.1.2

A primigravid patient 34 weeks' pregnant comes to see you in the antenatal clinic requesting a home birth.

A What is the approximate home birth rate in the UK? (1 mark)
B What are the advantages of a planned home birth? (8 marks)
C What are the two commonest indications for transfer to hospital for a woman planning a home birth? (2 marks)
D Give three examples of the risks of delivering at home. (4 marks)
E What local arrangements must be in place to support home births? (5 marks)

Key words in the question

- Primigravid, 34 weeks' pregnant, home birth.
- Home birth rate.
- Advantages.
- Two commonest indications, transfer to hospital.
- Risks.
- Local arrangements, support home births.

Essay plan

A
- Rate = 2%.

B
- Lower intervention, higher satisfaction.

C
- Failure to progress, epidural.

D
- Unexpected obstetric complications, maternal bleeding, fetal distress, flat baby.

E
- Local policies, transfer, contact senior support, ambulance involvement.

Suggested answer

A

The rate of home birth in the UK is approximately 2% (1).

B

There is good observational evidence to suggest that home birth is a safe option for many women (1). This evidence has also shown that there is a lower intervention rate in home birth. There is a reduction in induction of labour, augmentation, perineal trauma, including episiotomy, instrumental delivery and caesarean section (5).

There is higher maternal satisfaction due to an increased sense of control, empowerment and self-esteem (2).

C

The two commonest indications for transfer to hospital in planned home birth are slow progress in labour and patient request for analgesia, particularly epidural analgesia (2).

D

The main danger of a planned home birth is the risk of an unexpected and unpredictable obstetric emergency (1). This can include maternal haemorrhage, concerns regarding the fetus (presumed fetal distress) and a baby born in an unexpectedly poor condition (3).

E

Local policies should be in place to support home births (1).

There should be arrangements to transfer the woman in an emergency to the most appropriate place, e.g. the obstetric labour ward, not the accident and emergency department (1).

There should be an arrangement to contact the most senior obstetrician on the labour ward for obstetric problems (1) and the senior resident paediatrician in the case of a neonatal problem (1).

These agreements have to be implemented in cooperation with the local ambulance services, to facilitate such transfers in a timely manner to the most appropriate destination (1).

Further reading

Royal College of Obstetricians and Gynaecologists and Royal College of Midwives. *Home Births*. Joint Statement No. 2. London: RCOG, April 2007.

2.6.1.3

3 A 26-year-old primigravida at 30 weeks' gestation presents to the antenatal clinic with widespread itching.

A Describe initial management. (6 marks)

B A diagnosis of obstetric cholestasis (OC) is made. How should the rest of her pregnancy be managed? (10 marks)

C How should she be managed in the postnatal period? (4 marks)

Key words in the question

- 26-year-old, 30 weeks' gestation, itching.
- Initial management.
- OC, pregnancy, managed.
- Managed, postnatal period.

Essay plan

A
- Consider differential diagnosis and establish diagnosis.
- Check fetal well-being.

B
- Combined medical antenatal care.
- Symptomatic relief of mother and monitoring of fetus.
- Timing of delivery.

C
- Explain recurrence risk.
- Contraceptive advice.
- Ensure liver function returns to normal.

Suggested answer

A

A detailed history of the duration of itching, at what time of the day or night it is worst, and which part of the body is most affected should be elicited.

Other causes of itching such as infections, drug allergies, pruritus of pregnancy and exacerbation of dermatological conditions such as eczema should be excluded.

A family history of obstetric cholestasis (OC) or any other evidence of cholestasis such as dark urine or pale stools should be sought (4).

The woman is examined for any rashes and blood taken for liver function and bile acids.

Assessment of the fetus by cardiotocography and ultrasound should be carried out (2).

B

The diagnosis and its implications for the pregnancy should be explained to the woman.

The management of OC should include input from a hepatologist if possible, or in a medical antenatal clinic.

An ultrasound scan of the liver and serology for hepatitis should be arranged to exclude other causes of abnormal liver function results (3).

The woman may be given topical emollients for symptomatic relief (1).

Ursodeoxycholic acid can be prescribed to enhance bile acid clearance, although there is little evidence that it is effective (1).

Vitamin K should be prescribed at 10 mg per day orally to reduce the risk of haemorrhage in both mother and baby (1).

The woman should be given steroids parenterally for enhancing fetal lung maturity, as there is a spontaneous or iatrogenic risk of prematurity (1).

The monitoring of liver function and bile acids should be done as per local protocol (1).

Regular assessment of fetal well-being should be performed. There is no evidence that a premature delivery decreases the risk of stillbirth (1).

Timing of delivery must be discussed with the patient after weighing up the risks of iatrogenic prematurity versus the risk of sudden intrauterine death (1).

C

The woman should be reassured that there will be no long-term sequelae for her or her baby from OC (1).

She should be advised that there is a high recurrence rate of this condition in future pregnancies (1).

Liver function tests should be checked about 10 days after delivery to ensure that they have returned to normal (1).

Contraceptive advice must include the avoidance of the combined oral contraceptive pill (1).

Further reading

Royal College of Obstetricians and Gynaecologists. *Obstetric Cholestasis*. Green-Top Guideline No. 43. London: RCOG, January 2006.

2 **2.6.1.4**

A What is female genital mutilation (FGM)? Outline the different types. (5 marks)

B A patient with FGM books for antenatal care at 12 weeks' gestation in her first pregnancy. Outline appropriate antenatal and delivery management. (7 marks)

C If this woman has type 3 FGM, what are the possible obstetric complications? (7 marks)

D Following delivery she requests reinfibulation. What would you do? (1 mark)

Key words in the question

- Female genital mutilation, different types.
- Antenatal care, 12 weeks, antenatal and delivery management.
- Type 3 FGM, obstetric complications.
- Reinfibulation.

Essay plan

A
- Definition. Types 1–4.

B
- Explain possible adverse effects and assess extent of FGM.
- Nutrition, risk UTIs, defibulation before 20 weeks (ideally).
- Psychosexual counselling.

C
- Obstructed labour, perineal tears, higher CS rate, postpartum haemorrhage, postnatal wound infection.
- Maternal and neonatal morbidity and mortality.

D
- More scarring with reinfibulation – also illegal. Repair tears, episiotomy.

Suggested answer

A

Female genital mutilation (FGM) is defined as partial or complete removal of the female external genitalia for non-medical reasons (1). There are four types. Type 1 involves excision of the prepuce with or without excision of part or all of the clitoris (1). Type 2 is excision of the clitoris with partial or total excision of the labia minora (1). Type 3 is excision of part or all of the external genitalia and stitching or narrowing of the vaginal opening (infibulation) (1). Type 4 FGM is unclassified – it includes pricking, piercing, incising, stretching or scraping of the clitoris and/or labia and introduction of corrosive substances into the vagina to cause tightening and narrowing (1).

B

This patient should be treated with kindness and sympathy and in a non-judgemental way (1). I would explain that FGM may cause problems at delivery and offer to gently inspect and assess the extent of her FGM (1). If the urinary meatus is visible and if two fingers can be inserted into the vagina without discomfort, the mutilation is unlikely to cause major problems at delivery. Digital assessment is not always needed, as physical appearance may provide the reassurance required (1). I would advise the patient about the importance of good nutrition, as some women with FGM try to limit the size of the baby by cutting down on food, hoping that a smaller baby will result in an easier birth (1). I would explain that she is more likely to develop urinary tract and vaginal infections and arrange regular urine testing (1). I would offer defibulation before 20 weeks' gestation (1). [This ensures the scar is fully healed before labour, and the introitus is adequate for vaginal examination and prevents excessive blood loss at delivery. It also permits application of a fetal scalp electrode and fetal blood sampling in labour if necessary.] She should be offered psychosexual counselling in conjunction with her partner (1).

C

Possible obstetric complications of type 3 FGM include prolonged or obstructed labour (1), an increase in the number of perineal tears and epi-siotomies (1), a higher caesarean section rate (1), an increased risk of post-partum haemorrhage (1), an increased incidence of postnatal wound infection (1), possible maternal death from obstructed labour, with or without post-partum haemorrhage (1), and increased neonatal morbidity (from hypoxia) and death (1).

D

I would explain that reinfibulation causes more scarring and has deleterious effects on subsequent sexual and reproductive health. I would refuse to reinfibulate because it is illegal to do so in the UK (1) (FGM Act 2003). [However, it is important to repair any lacerations sufficiently to oppose raw edges and control bleeding and not intentionally to make the vaginal opening tighter.]

Further reading

Rashid M, Rashid MH. Obstetric management of women with female genital mutilation. *The Obstetrician and Gynaecologist* 2007; **9**: 95–101.

Royal College of Obstetricians and Gynaecologists. *Female Genital Muti-lation*. Statement No. 3. London: RCOG, May 2003.

Paper 2

2.6.2.1

Jane, a 15-year-old girl, attends a party and has unprotected sex with a 16-year-old, James, whom she knows from school. Jane comes from a strict Catholic background. She attends the accident and emergency department the next day requesting emergency contraception. You are the gynaecology doctor on call.

A Outline what further information you would need in order to counsel and treat this girl. (7 marks)

B Discuss the criteria, in relation to this case, which need to be met to deem someone less than 16 years of age 'Fraser ruling competent'. (4 marks)

C Would you do anything differently if Jane were aged 13 years or less? Is there an ethical dilemma to maintain confidentiality? (5 marks)

D The emergency contraception fails and Jane attends the outpatient clinic six weeks later requesting termination of pregnancy. She comes with her 17-year-old sister, who offers to sign the consent form for Jane, as their parents remain unaware of the pregnancy. What do you do? (4 marks)

Key words in the question

- 15-year-old, unprotected sex, emergency contraception.
- Information, counsel and treat.
- Criteria, 'Fraser ruling competent'.
- Differently, 13 years, ethical dilemma, confidentiality.
- Termination of pregnancy, 17-year-old sister, parents unaware.

Essay plan

A
- History – menstrual, sexual, consensual intercourse.
- Confidentiality.

B
- Lord Fraser's four criteria.

C
- Yes – child protection and social services.
- Break confidentiality if child deemed 'at risk'.

D
- Establish whether Jane is able to consent.
- If not, sister cannot consent as not next of kin.

Suggested answer

A
In this situation I would need to take a history from Jane (1).

I would establish her menstrual cycle and pattern and her last menstrual period (LMP) (1).

Jane's sexual history needs to be explored, in particular whether this was her only episode of unprotected intercourse in this menstrual cycle, to establish the correct emergency contraceptive to use [oral progestogen or intrauterine device] (2).

Discussion should take place with Jane to establish whether consent for sexual intercourse was obtained, and signs of coercion and abuse should be looked for (2).

Confidentiality should be maintained (1).

B

Lord Fraser ruled in 1985 that a doctor could give contraceptive advice or treatment if the following criteria were met.

The girl must be mature enough to understand the advice given and the implications of treatment (1).

She would be likely to continue or begin to have sex (1).

An attempt had been made by the doctor to encourage the girl to involve her parents (1).

The girl's health would suffer without treatment or advice and it was in the girl's best interests for the doctor to give contraceptive advice or treatment (1).

C

If Jane were 13 years old or less, I would discuss the case with the NHS Trust's lead for child protection. As a result, it is likely that this case would be reported to children's social services (2).

The potential for an ethical dilemma occurs if Jane does not wish to involve the lead for child protection and/or social services. However, if the risk to Jane is deemed serious enough, e.g. there is a high risk of an abusive relationship, then this overrides her right to privacy (2).

Local child protection protocols should be followed (1).

D

Jane needs to be assessed to see whether she is competent to give consent (1).

If she can understand the implications of the treatment, then she should be allowed to sign her own consent form (1).

If Jane is deemed unable to give consent, then the only people who can agree to the procedure on her behalf are those with parental responsibility or a court. Her 17-year-old sister cannot consent on Jane's behalf (2).

Further reading

Fleming CF. Young people and the Fraser guidelines: confidentiality and consent. *The Obstetrician and Gynaecologist* 2006; 8: 235–9.

2.6.2.2

A Outline the surgical options for the treatment of stress urinary incontinence (SUI). (5 marks)

B Using your answer to A, discuss the success rates and main complications for each procedure. (15 marks)

Key words in the question

A
- Outline, surgical, SUI.

B
- Discuss, success rates, main complications, each procedure.

Essay plan

A

- Main options for surgical treatment of SUI, including colposuspension, slings, injections and artificial sphincters.
- Success rates and complications for each.

Suggested answer

A

The main techniques used to treat stress urinary incontinence (SUI) are: open retropubic procedures, such as Burch colposuspension and laparoscopic colposuspension; sling procedures (open and minimally invasive); periurethral bulking agents; and artificial sphincters (5).

B

The success rate of Burch colposuspension is approximately 85% at one year, dropping to 70% by five years. The main complications of this procedure include voiding disorder, at an incidence of approximately 10%; de novo detrusor overactivity, at approximately 17%; and genitourinary prolapse (particularly rectocele and enterocele), at about 14% (4).

Laparoscopic colposuspension has the advantage over open colposuspension of avoiding a large incision, and this gives a shorter hospital stay. Recent trials have shown laparoscopic colposuspension to have a poorer outcome compared with open colposuspension. The complications are similar to those seen with open colposuspension (2).

Sling procedures can be divided into open and minimally invasive. Slings have a continence rate of approximately 80%, with a further 10% improved. Minimally invasive retropubic slings using a 'bottom-up' technique (such as tension-free vaginal tape – TVT) are currently recommended by the National Institute for Health and Clinical Excellence (NICE) and have the main complications of bladder perforation, at up to 9%; de novo detrusor overactivity, at up to 5%; and an approximately 3% chance of voiding disorder. Open slings have complications of voiding disorder at 10%, detrusor overactivity at 14%, and tape erosion (when synthetic materials are used) of approximately 9% (4).

Injectable bulking agents have a lower success rate than other procedures, with a short-term continence rate of 48% and an improvement rate of approximately 76%. There is a continued decline in continence rates over time but this procedure has a low morbidity and may be useful in the patient who is unfit for major surgery or when other procedures have failed (3).

Artificial sphincters can be successful (up to 90% success quoted) after previous surgery but have a high morbidity, including a reoperation rate of approximately 17% (2).

Further reading

Johnson H, Slack M. Evidence-based management of stress urinary incontinence. *The Obstetrician and Gynaecologist* 2005; 7: 159–65.

National Institute for Health and Clinical Excellence. The Management of Urinary Incontinence in Women. Clinical Guideline No. 40. London: NICE, October 2006.

Royal College of Obstetricians and Gynaecologists. *Surgical Treatment of Urodynamic Stress Incontinence*. Green-Top Guideline No. 35. London: RCOG, October 2003.

2.6.2.3

A 27-year-old, nulliparous woman is referred to the gynaecology outpatient department with symptoms strongly suggestive of endometriosis.

A What clinical features are typically associated with endometriosis? (6 marks)

B How can endometriosis be definitively diagnosed? (1 mark)

C Discuss the medical treatment options available if this patient has endometriosis-associated pain? (5 marks)

D What surgical options are available for treating endometriosis? (6 marks)

E If this patient has minimal–mild endometriosis and wishes to conceive, outline your management. (2 marks)

Key words in the question

- 27-year-old, nulliparous, endometriosis.
- Clinical features.
- Definitively diagnosed.
- Medical treatment options, endometriosis-associated pain.
- Surgical options.
- Minimal–mild endometriosis, conceive, management.

Essay plan

A
- Symptoms and signs.

B
- Diagnostic laparoscopy.

C
- NSAIDs, hormonal therapy – COCP, gestrinone, MPA, GnRHa.
- LNG–IUS.

D
- Laparoscopy.
- Laparotomy.

E
- Laparoscopy with ablation +/− adhesiolysis.

Suggested answer

A

The typical clinical features associated with endometriosis include severe dysmenorrhoea, deep dyspareunia, chronic pelvic pain, infertility, cyclical or perimenstrual symptoms and dyschezia. Signs include pelvic tenderness, a fixed retroverted uterus and tender uterosacral ligaments (6).

B

Visual inspection of the pelvis at laparoscopy is the gold standard for diagnosing endometriosis (1).

C

Medical treatment for endometriosis-associated pain includes non-steroidal anti-inflammatory drugs (NSAIDs) (although evidence of effectiveness is inconclusive). Suppression of ovarian function for six months reduces endometriosis-associated pain. Hormonal drugs such as the combined oral contraceptive pill (COCP), gestrinone, danazol, medroxyprogesterone acetate and gonadotrophin-releasing hormone (GnRH) agonists are equally effective. Duration of therapy is limited for some drugs and the adverse-effect profiles differ. The COCP and Depo-Provera can be used long term, but GnRH agonist use is usually restricted to six months due to the risk of osteoporosis. However, GnRH agonists with 'add-back' therapy, e.g. tibolone, protect against loss of bone mineral density, may be safely used and are effective for up to at least two years.

A levonorgestrel-containing intrauterine system (Mirena) appears to reduce endometriosis-associated pain (5).

D

The optimum surgical treatment for endometriosis-associated pain is laparoscopy with excision/ablation of endometriotic deposits. However, some women fail to respond to surgical treatment because of incomplete excision, because of postoperative disease recurrence or because some of their pain was not due to endometriosis in the first place. If a hysterectomy is performed, all visible endometriotic tissue should be removed at the same time. Bilateral salpingo-oophorectomy (BSO) may improve pain relief and reduce the chance of the patient requiring future surgery. Hormone replacement therapy (HRT) is recommended after BSO in young women, although the ideal regime is unclear. Giving combined oestrogen and progestogen protects against the unopposed action of oestrogen on any residual disease (6).

E

Medical treatment is unsuccessful in improving fertility in minimal–mild endometriosis. Laparoscopy with ablation of endometriotic lesions plus adhesiolysis (if necessary) improves fertility. Medical treatment after surgery appears not to improve pregnancy rates (2).

Further reading

Royal College of Obstetricians and Gynaecologists. *The Investigation and Management of Endometriosis*. Green-Top Guideline No. 24. London: RCOG, October 2006.

2.6.2.4

A 15-year-old girl presents with delayed pubertal development. Chromosomal investigations reveal Turner syndrome.

A Outline your principles of management. (8 marks)

B Justify your management through adolescence. (6 marks)

C Justify your management through adult life. (6 marks)

Key words in the question

- 15-year-old, delayed pubertal development, Turner syndrome.
- Principles of management.
- Management, adolescence.
- Management, adult life.

Essay plan

A
- Break news to patient.
- Psychological support.
- Medical management.

B
- Hormonal replacement.
- Place of growth hormone.

C
- Fertility issues.
- Medical surveillance.
- HRT.

Suggested answer

A

Breaking the news of Turner syndrome to a young girl can be traumatic for her and her family and challenging for the doctor (1). This information should be given to the patient in the presence of her mother or next of kin, who can support her through this difficult time (1). She should be informed that although this is a genetic condition (45XO), she is likely to have a normal lifespan (1).

Turner syndrome is not inherited genetically. The patient should be offered psychological support, and she should be advised to get in touch with other patients with this condition through support groups such as the Turner Syndrome Support Society (2).

She should be referred to a physician for a medical review, as patients with Turner syndrome are at higher risk of cardiac problems such as coarctation of the aorta and/or a bicuspid aortic valve, hypertension secondary to cardiac or renal problems, and type 2 diabetes (1).

Hormone replacement therapy (HRT) will be required (1).

Although she will be infertile, she may be able to have a child through oocyte donation (1).

B

The patient should be informed that the average adult height of women with Turner syndrome is approximately 145 cm (1). Growth hormone helps to increase the height slightly but only if used early in teenage life (1). The timing and benefits of this should be discussed with an endocrinologist (1).

Oestrogen replacement is needed to help the development of the breasts and her secondary sexual characteristics (2). The best form of treatment at this stage is the combined oral contraceptive pill, as it is more socially acceptable in this age group than HRT (1).

C

The patient should be kept under medical surveillance because of the higher risks of hypertension secondary to renal problems and because of the potential to develop type 2 diabetes and its sequelae (2).

She will require referral to a specialist fertility centre when and if she wishes to have children. This will necessitate oocyte donation and hormonal support, usually in the form of sequential HRT to mimic the natural hormonal cycles (3).

She should be advised to continue with HRT until about the age of 50 years in order to try to minimize the risks of osteoporosis (1).

Further reading

Ashraf M, Jayawickrama NS, Bowen-Simpkins P. Premature ovarian failure due to an unbalanced translocation on the X chromosome. *British Journal of Obstetrics and Gynaecology* 2001; **108**: 230–2.

Bhattacharya S, Hamilton M. *Management of Infertility for the MRCOG and Beyond*. London: RCOG Press, 2006: 97–113.

Index